CHARLOTTE LIBOV is the award-winning co-author of *50 Essential Things to Do When the Doctor Says It's Heart Disease*, *The Woman's Heart Book*, and the upcoming *Conquering the Odds: A Woman's Guide to Beating Her Risk Factors*. She lectures on women's health issues, frequently appears on radio and television, and her articles have appeared in the *New York Times*. Ms. Libov has an M.S. in mental health counseling from the University of Oregon, and lives in Bethlehem, Connecticut.

MIGRAINE

50 ESSENTIAL THINGS TO DO

Charlotte Libov

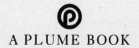

A PLUME BOOK

PLUME
Published by the Penguin Group
Penguin Putnam Inc., 375 Hudson Street, New York, New York 10014, U.S.A.
Penguin Books Ltd, 27 Wrights Lane, London W8 5TZ, England
Penguin Books Australia Ltd, Ringwood, Victoria, Australia
Penguin Books Canada Ltd, 10 Alcorn Avenue, Toronto, Ontario, Canada M4V 3B2
Penguin Books (N.Z.) Ltd, 182–190 Wairau Road, Auckland 10, New Zealand

Penguin Books Ltd, Registered Offices: Harmondsworth, Middlesex, England

First published by Plume, an imprint of Dutton NAL,
a member of Penguin Putnam Inc.

First Printing, November, 1998
10 9 8 7 6 5 4 3 2 1

 REGISTERED TRADEMARK—MARCA REGISTRADA

LIBRARY OF CONGRESS CATALOGING-IN-PUBLICATION DATA
Libov, Charlotte.
Migraine: 50 essential things to do / Charlotte Libov.
p.   cm.
Includes index.
ISBN 0-452-27726-4
1. Migraine—Popular works.   I. Title.
RC392.L52   1998
616.8'57—dc21   98-4235
                                    CIP

Printed in the United States of America
Set in Caslon 540
Designed by Julian Hamer

A NOTE TO THE READER

The ideas, procedures, and suggestions contained in this book are not intended as a substitute for medical treatment by a physician. The reader should regularly consult a physician in matters relating to health.

*This book is dedicated
with all my love to my mother*

CONTENTS

ACKNOWLEDGMENTS

So many people are instrumental in the writing of a book, it is difficult to acknowledge all of their contributions. However, for their specific help in this book, I would like to thank the following experts who gave generously of their time and expertise. They include: Roger Cady, M.D.; Donald J. Delessio, M.D.; R. Merle Diamond, M.D.; Seymour Diamond, M.D.; R. Michael Gallagher, D.O.; Elizabeth Loder, M.D.; Michael G. McKee, Ph.D.; Robert S. Kunkel, M.D.; Robert W. Rosum, RPH, M.S.; Fred D. Sheftell, M.D.; Ramesh Sogol, M.D.; Glen Soloman, M.D.; Grace Steere, M.D.; Marla Tobin, M.D.; and Alexander Mauskop, M.D.

Additionally, I would like to thank Michael John Coleman, executive director of Migraine Awareness Group: A National Organization for Migraineurs (M.A.G.N.U.M), The American Association for the Study of Headache, the American Council for Headache Education (ACHE), the National Headache Foundation, and the Center for the Advancement of Health.

I am also greatly indebted to the migraine sufferers I've

met on the on-line services CompuServe and America Online, for their friendship, encouragement, and their generosity in being willing to share their stories in the hope of helping others.

Also, I wish to thank my literary agent, Carole Abel, my editor, Jennifer Moore, for her expertise and patience, and of course, Terry Montlick, my partner, for his enthusiasm and support.

PART ONE

UNDERSTANDING MIGRAINE

#1

EMPOWER YOURSELF

This book is designed to explore the new thinking about migraine, explore new treatments for it, and encourage both you, the migraine sufferer, and your friends, coworkers, and families to view your migraines in a different light.

In this book, you'll learn that, contrary to past belief, migraine is a neurological disease, not a psychological problem. You'll learn about treatments that use drugs; other therapies; lifestyle modifications; and the new wave of activism designed to insure the rights of migraineurs.

There's a wealth of information in this book, but it's up to you to put these steps into practice. This isn't easy, especially when you're dealing with a chronic, disabling disease that causes bouts of excruciating pain followed by days spent drained and exhausted. But to get effective care, you must take an active role in learning about migraines and determining what changes you need to make.

Because migraines tend to run in families, sufferers too often have learned from their parents or grandparents to just deal with their attacks by enduring them. But that was in the old days, when nothing much could be done. That is no longer the case. There are new, effective treatments, but you must be willing to give them a try.

Bear in mind that migraine is often misdiagnosed. There is much confusion about what distinguishes migraine from other types of headaches. To get the proper treatment, you must first be properly diagnosed. To do this, you need to learn about migraine, pay attention to your symptoms, and, if necessary, seek the right professional help.

Since there are many more treatments available now than there used to be, you need to stay current. Furthermore, because of the way the health care system has changed, you must be your own health care advocate and make sure you're getting the coverage you're entitled to.

Finding relief from your migraines may also involve speaking up. In the old days, many migraineurs sought to hide their ailment because they were afraid of seeming weak. As you read through this book, you may realize that certain elements of your work place, your environment, or your lifestyle trigger your migraines. Calling attention to themselves is something that most migraineurs are not comfortable doing, but it may be necessary.

Obviously, this puts the responsibility for dealing with your migraines on you, but that's also liberating. Because migraine is increasingly being recognized as a neurological disease, you no longer need to live with the uneasy feeling that you brought this ailment upon yourself.

FOR MEN ONLY

Migraines occur far more often in women than men. But millions of men are also affected. However, because migraine is characterized as a "woman's disease," many men hide their affliction.

Furthermore, because migraine is associated with women, men tend to assume their headaches are "sinus" headaches, hangovers, or some other type of headache malady. With the advent of new prescription drugs, advertising of migraine treatments is increasing, but because of the demographics these ads tend to feature women.

Many men may not realize they have migraine and, if they do, they may assume there aren't effective treatments for it. Or they may treat their attacks with over-the-counter medications, which may be ineffective and lead to a worse headache problem. Or they may borrow medication from their friends or from their wives, which is unwise. They may self-medicate themselves by turning to alcohol, which has its obvious problems as well.

In addition, because migraine is considered a woman's problem, men may fear that they'll be passed over for promotions because of the myth that migraines are caused by stress, or that if they call in sick, they won't be believed. They may be ashamed to be open about their pain to their families because they don't want to seem weak.

Accepting these myths only compounds them. If you are a man who suffers from migraines, take charge. You have a biological disease, not an emotional weakness for which you should feel ashamed. Migraine treatments work for both men and women.

#2

Learn the Toll Migraine Takes

Of all the medical ailments that cause great pain and suffering, migraine is one of the most common, and one of the most misunderstood.

In ancient times, migraines were ascribed to evil spirits. As the centuries progressed, drastic measures were prescribed for migraine sufferers, including purging, bloodletting, and even drilling holes in the head. That migraine sufferers eagerly sought such harrowing treatments is proof of how painful and frightening this disease can be.

Over the centuries, the view of migraine has changed. It was once considered a psychological disorder, probably brought on by stress; doctors now know that migraine is a disease, as legitimate a medical condition as cancer, diabetes, or heart disease. In addition, migraine was once viewed simply as severe headaches; between attacks, the migraineur was assumed to be fine. Now, experts view migraine more broadly as a disease that affects the entire body. People who get migraines are also at increased risk for other conditions, including depression, panic attacks, and even stroke.

In fact, it's only now being recognized how complex a disease migraine is. Migraineurs often differ from each other widely. They may share certain patterns of pain in common, but often that's where the similarity ends. This is what makes treating migraine so challenging, and sometimes so frustrating.

Migraine is also a very common disease. It's estimated that nearly fifteen million Americans suffer from agonizing migraines, according to a survey published in the *Journal of the American Medical Association*. That survey estimated that 8.7 million women and 6.2 million men suffer from this problem. Of this number, 3.4 million women and 1.1 million men experience one or more attacks per month. Women between the ages of thirty and forty-nine have the most attacks—often so severe that sufferers are forced to seek help at an emergency room.

But statistics don't begin to express the profound despair many migraineurs suffer. Consider what migraineurs told a Gallup poll about how migraine impacts their daily lives:

- Thirty-five percent have found the pain of an attack so excruciating that, during it, they've wished they were dead.
- Many rated the pain of their migraine as more severe than childbirth, a broken bone, arthritis, or being seriously injured or badly burned.
- Thirty-nine percent said that migraine had hampered their careers, their earnings, or their educational pursuits.
- Nearly three quarters said that migraine interfered with at least one important aspect of their lives.

But, despite these serious ramifications, about half of the survey participants responded that their family and friends don't understand how serious and painful a problem migraine is. Research done by Robert Smith, M.D., founder of the Headache Center at the University of Cincinnati, underscores the profound impact that migraine exacts from family and relationships. According to his survey, reported in 1998, 18 percent of his participants directly attributed their divorce to migraine. About a quarter of those surveyed blamed migraine for interfering with their sexual relations, others said migraine had left their families feeling frustrated and resentful and 10 percent said it caused them to seek marital counseling.

These are the facts which you can use to demonstrate to others, and to yourself, about the toll that migraine takes.

#3

LEARN WHAT MIGRAINE IS— AND ISN'T

The first thing you need to know is whether or not you indeed get migraine headaches. This is a very relevant question. You may be surprised to learn how many different types of headaches there are. In fact, the International Headache Society divides headaches into thirteen major classifications with sixty-six subdivisions, as well as a catchall category, "nonclassifiable headaches." This makes headache a very complicated subject medically.

Part of the confusion is due to the way headache is portrayed in the media. The Food and Drug Administration (FDA) dictates that, in order for a company to advertise a product as a migraine reliever, that product must be shown to actually relieve migraines. In the absence of such proof, the ads for most pain relievers generalize; they may show sufferers experiencing classic migraine signs, but since the word *migraine* can't be used, these symptoms are attributed to "sinus" or "tension-type" headaches. As a result, people often think that if their head pain is mild, it's a sinus or tension headache and, if it's severe, it's migraine.

Too often, articles and television reports on headache lump different types together, giving the impression that they are similar. But migraines are different from other types of headache. As the understanding of migraine has grown, it's become evident that migraines have different causes from other types of headaches, and different treatments as well. Some medications intended for tension headache don't relieve migraine, and vice versa. Increasingly, an accurate diagnosis is essential for effectively treating migraine.

The most common forms of headaches fall into four major categories. There are two types of migraine: migraine with aura and migraine without aura. You may also hear these two called classic migraine and common migraine, respectively. The other most common types of headache are tension and cluster headaches.

More detailed descriptions of migraine follow in the next chapter, but here's a brief look at the most common types of headache.

THE MOST COMMON TYPES OF MIGRAINE

Migraine without Aura (Common Migraine)
This is defined as a recurring headache, usually throbbing and severe, that is often accompanied by nausea and vomiting, as well as extreme sensitivity to light, sound, or motion. Although sufferers don't experience aura, they may have a vague premonition of an impending attack, which is known as a prodrome.

Migraine with Aura (Classic Migraine)
Those with this type of headache suffer from neurological symptoms, which usually include flashing lights or patterns, losing part of their visual field, hallucinations in hearing or

smell, or possibly numbness or tingling in their arms or legs. These symptoms are followed about thirty minutes later by severe head pain and possibly gastrointestinal symptoms like nausea and vomiting.

OTHER TYPES OF MIGRAINE

These are types of migraine that are less common than the two just described, but you need to know about them because they are often misdiagnosed.

Migraine Equivalents
This is a type of migraine that does not involve a headache. However, it can cause either the visual symptoms of migraine with aura or the gastrointestinal symptoms associated with migraine with or without aura. As with migraine, the symptoms may last for hours and reoccur. Migraine equivalents are not more serious than the more common forms of migraine, but sufferers can go for years without being properly diagnosed and treated. Sufferers of this condition usually have a personal or family history of migraine.

Basilar Migraine
This type of migraine is characterized by confusion, unsteadiness, dizziness, slurring of speech, ringing in the ears, and numbness of the tongue and lips. Visual disturbances can include blurriness, seeing flashes, graying of vision, or total loss of vision. Sufferers can appear to be in a dreamlike state that can progress into loss of consciousness and even coma. Most people with this type of migraine also experience headache, nausea, and vomiting. Seizures are also possible. This rare type of migraine usually occurs first in childhood or adolescence, or in people in their twenties and thirties, although it is possible for it to begin in people over the age of fifty. This condition can be mistaken for drunkenness or a mental disorder.

Hemiplegic Migraine

This type of migraine causes symptoms that resemble stroke and, indeed, in rare cases, can even result in a migraine-related stroke. The major characteristic of this type of migraine is paralysis, which usually spreads slowly down one side of the body. Visual disturbances or aura can occur, and sufferers may also have difficulty speaking. These symptoms are usually followed by a severe, throbbing headache, nausea, and vomiting; and sensitivity to light and sound are also common. Another form of this ailment is known as familial hemiplegic migraine, meaning that the disease is inherited.

Retinal Migraine

Also known as ocular migraine, this condition occurs in one out of every two hundred migraine sufferers; they may or may not have previously experienced auras. It is characterized by blindness or blurred vision in one eye. Headache may precede, follow, or accompany this visual disturbance. The visual problems usually last a few minutes but can last longer and even, although rarely, become permanent.

Ophthalmoplegic Migraine

This exceedingly rare type of migraine begins as a headache followed by double vision which can persist for up to several days. The most telling symptom of this type of migraine is a dilated pupil on one side, and the inability to move the eye to see up or down.

OTHER TYPES OF HEADACHES

Tension Headaches

Although migraines with and without aura are common, tension headaches are even more so. In fact, they are the most common form of headache. Sufferers often describe the pain as feeling as though a tight band is encircling their head. These headaches vary in severity from mild to moderate, and they can last for hours, days, or even longer. Although the pain may be less severe than a migraine, these headaches can be very frequent and debilitating.

Cluster Headaches

These severe headaches are more rare than migraines. Unlike migraines, which are more common in women, cluster headaches usually occur in men. They are characterized by sharp, penetrating pain that can be prolonged or brief and can occur once, twice, or up to ten times a day. They can continue for months and then disappear, only to reoccur later. Cluster headaches are usually accompanied by a stuffy or runny nose and a watering eye. But even though men usually get cluster headaches, there is one type, known as "chronic paroxysmal hemicrania," which occurs more often in middle-aged women.

Fortunately, there is medication available for men and women who suffer from cluster headaches, but most of these drugs are used specifically for this type of headache. Oxygen is also sometimes used. If you suspect cluster headache is your problem, see a headache specialist or doctor experienced in treating them.

Chronic Daily Headache (CDH)

The head pain associated with the problem known as Chronic Daily Headache may be less severe than migraine, but can be just as draining because it is pain which occurs very frequently, even daily. In fact, CDH is defined as headaches which occur more often than 180 days a year.

CDH usually manifests itself as a tightness or pressure which may occur on both sides of the head. When migraines evolve into this type of headache problem, it is known as "transformed migraine." CDH can also occur in those who suffer from tension headaches or following an injury.

Transformed Migraine

If you previously experienced distinct migraine attacks but now find yourself beset with them daily or almost every day, you may be suffering from this form of CDH. These are the characteristics of this problem:

- You experience headache more than 15 days a month or 180 days a year
- You previously experienced distinct migraine attacks
- Your headaches resemble migraine attacks
- If you're a woman, your headaches may grow worse in accordance with your menstrual cycle
- You may also experience depression, anxiety, or stress

An estimated 80 percent of cases of CDH, both the transformed migraine and nonmigraine type, is believed to be caused by overuse of over-the-counter and prescription drugs. See Chapter 25 for more on this very important topic.

#4

ANSWER THESE TEN QUESTIONS

As you know, migraine is so common, there's even a special name for the people who suffer from them. They're called migraineurs. Are you a migraineur? Answer these next ten questions to find out. Answer them even if you're convinced you're a migraineur. You'll gain information that you can use to improve your condition.

1. HOW OLD WERE YOU WHEN YOUR HEADACHES STARTED?

Typically the first one occurs between six and twenty-five years of age. They can begin later, but if you're in your fifties and you've just begun experiencing severe headaches, your doctor will want to rule out other causes. Cluster headaches most often begin in the thirties and forties. For women, a first migraine can occur when one begins menstruating, is pregnant, or is approaching menopause.

2. How often do you get them?

As with everything related to migraine, the main rule is that
there isn't a rule. Some people may experience only one attack
in their whole lifetime, while others may suffer several attacks
a week. On average, though, most migraine sufferers report one
or two attacks a month. Women who experience hormone-
related migraines find their attacks correlate with their menstrual cycle. It's rare for migraines to occur daily, so if you do
experience daily, or almost daily, headache, you may be suffering from CDH, a frustrating condition that can be brought on
by overuse of medication, even the over-the-counter kind.
There's more on this problem later in the book.

3. Where does the pain occur?

This is sometimes a telltale sign of migraine. Migraine pain is
usually experienced on only one side of the head; indeed, the
word *migraine* comes from the Greek word *hemikrania*, which
means "half a skull." Such pain can always occur on a certain
side or switch sides. But this is not a hard and fast rule; it's possible for the pain to be felt anywhere about the head
or neck.

4. How long does the pain last?

Typically, the period of intense pain from a migraine lasts from
four to twenty-four hours, although it can last up to forty-eight
hours. Migraines that last longer than that are referred to as sta-
tus migraines, which involve severe, unremitting migraine pain,
often with nausea and vomiting, that may require emergency
room treatment or even hospitalization.

5. WHAT DOES THE PAIN FEEL LIKE?

Migraines bring with them a particular type of head pain most often described as intense, violent, unbearable, pulsing, or throbbing. But that doesn't begin to tell the whole story. Here's how migraine sufferers describe it:

My migraines start in a dull way over one eye and continue down the back of my head. When I get them, I can't even sit in a chair that touches the back of my neck. I can't stand to look at the TV. Nothing I can do dulls the pain, which, by the second day, invades my skull and makes me feel just terrible.

—Marlene, a forty-one-year-old business administrator

When I'm in the midst of a migraine I have trouble moving my head, because of the pain. I'm nauseous, light hurts my eyes, I find any noise unbearable, and the pain is undescribable. It feels like my brain is being attacked.

—Bob, a forty-eight-year-old claims adjuster

6. IS THERE AN AURA OR "PRODROME"?

"Aura" is the name given to the one or more vivid visual or neurological symptoms experienced by some migraine sufferers. However, the belief that migraine must be accompanied by an aura is a myth. In fact, only 10 to 15 percent of migraine sufferers experience aura.

Auras manifest themselves shortly (an hour or two) before the head pain begins. The most common are visual occurrences, such as blind spots; bright, shimmering, or wavy lines; zigzag patterns; flashing lights; or distorted shapes. Less common sensations include burning, pricking, or the unpleasant feeling that something is crawling on one's skin. Still less commonly, speech problems can occur, such as slurring your speech or knowing what you want to say but being unable to find the words.

Some migraineurs who get auras, or even some who don't, may experience symptoms prior to an attack. This phenomenon is known as a preheadache or prodrome. These vague symptoms may include hunger, lack of appetite, drowsiness, depression, irritability, tension, and restlessness. On the other hand, sufferers of prodrome may become talkative, energetic, or infused with a sense of well-being. After the head pain subsides, particularly if it's been severe, there is sometimes a postheadache or postdrome period, leaving the sufferer feeling tired, listless, or depressed, sometimes with a tender scalp or achy muscles as well.

Migraine can be tricky. It's possible to experience the sensations of migraine, including visual disturbances, nausea, and vomiting, without the signature headache pain. Helen, for example, was perplexed by her repeated vomiting and nausea. Her symptoms corresponded to no known stomach ailment, and all her test results were negative. Finally a doctor discovered that she was suffering from a migraine equivalent—in her case, the gastrointestinal symptoms of a migraine, without the headache.

7. WHAT OTHER SYMPTOMS OCCUR?

Head pain is not the only symptom of a migraine. In fact, migraines used to be known as sick headaches, for a very good reason. Most migraine sufferers experience nausea along with their headaches, and many often are plagued with attacks of vomiting as well. Other symptoms can include sensitivity to light and sound, loss of appetite, diarrhea, dizziness, lightheadedness, chills, tremors, and cold hands and feet.

8. HOW DO YOU BEHAVE DURING AN ATTACK?

Typically, people suffering from migraine often find it impossible to carry on their normal activities. Often, they retreat to a quiet, dark room. They report that even the mildest physical activity or noise, such as the shutting of a door, will increase the pain tremendously. Even those who experience less severe attacks instinctively try to curb their normal activities.

9. DO OTHERS IN YOUR FAMILY GET MIGRAINES?

Most people who get migraines have relatives who get them as well. This can include parents or even grandparents. Most people can clearly recollect whether their family members suffer from migraine. But sometimes it's not that clear. For example, when Anne went to a headache clinic for migraine treatment, she was at a loss when she was asked about her family history. She recalled, though, that her father complained of double vision that his doctors were at a loss to explain. At the headache clinic, his eye problem was finally diagnosed as a migraine equivalent.

Here are some questions to ask yourself or your relatives:

- As you were growing up, do you recall a family member being sick much or some of the time?
- Did they exhibit any of the following symptoms or complain of:
  — Head pain that interfered with activities?
  — Nausea or vomiting?
  — Sensitivity to light or sound?
  — Seeing lights or shapes?
  — Having numbness or speech difficulty?

Knowing that you have family members who suffered from migraine can bring you closer to your own diagnosis. However, bear in mind that, although migraine tends to run in families, it doesn't always.

10. IF YOU'RE FEMALE, DO YOUR MIGRAINES PRECEDE OR COINCIDE WITH THE ONSET OF YOUR PERIOD?

If so, you may suffer from "menstrual migraines," migraines that are influenced by your hormones. You may have this problem if you began getting migraines when you first got your period or when you first became pregnant, or if your migraines disappeared during pregnancy, only to reappear later.

You can use the information you've gleaned from these questions in formulating your own migraine management plan or in working on one with your doctor.

#5

KEEP AN OPEN MIND

If you've only recently begun getting migraines, you may be eager to find help. But many chronic migraine sufferers already feel like they've tried everything.

This feeling is compounded if migraines run in your family and you've grown up seeing your relatives suffer helplessly. You may have watched your mother take to her bed, or you were shooed away from your father's shut study door. You may have seen your parents gulping too many pills, or stoically soldiering on, determined to ignore the pain, no matter what. They may have passed their habits and attitudes down to you. This is unfortunate, because it is now possible to eliminate much of this suffering. Yet old attitudes persist. So as you work your way through this book, keep an open mind.

On the other hand, be realistic. Tremendous strides have been made in treating migraines, but it's still best considered a manageable disease, not a curable one. Indeed, migraine sufferers who go from doctor to doctor fruitlessly seeking a "cure" are the ones who become the most frustrated. Much more can be done now than ever before, but having realistic expectations is the key to true relief.

"The vast majority of people who experience severe headaches who are very happy with their medical care are not those who are free of headaches. But they are those who know what to expect and how to handle their headaches. That's the important factor," notes Dr. R. Michael Gallagher, director of the University Headache Center in Moorestown, New Jersey.

#6

EXPLORE THE CAUSES OF MIGRAINE

Despite the strides made in migraine treatment, doctors still don't fully understand why migraines occur. Many factors can bring them on, even some that may not yet have been identified. If you're not prone to migraines, you may get headaches, but nothing—no matter what you do—will produce a migraine.

Why should you concern yourself with the biology of what causes migraine? First, learning about the biology will free you from any lingering misconceptions you may have that migraine is "all in your head" or that you are somehow to blame for your migraines. Second, learning how complicated this condition is will help you understand the basis of many of the treatments, so you may become more interested in giving them an appropriate trial or undertaking difficult lifestyle changes.

Research shows that migraine is a disease with strong genetic links. Various studies have found that a child has as much as a 40 percent chance of developing migraine if one parent is a migraine sufferer, a 75 percent chance if both parents are, and a 20 percent chance if a relative is. Furthermore, twin studies have found consistently higher rates of migraine among identical twins.

Unfortunately, the genetics of migraine is not simple. There is no evidence that a single gene causes this disease. Rather, it's likely that several genes interact with each other. These genes also apparently act together with environmental factors. So it's thought, for example, that you can inherit genes that make you prone to migraines which are then triggered by certain factors, such as particular foods, odors, or changes in the weather.

It's believed that inheriting such a genetic makeup makes a person susceptible to migraine, but does not mean that they definitely will develop it. An exception is the rare type of migraine known as familial hemiplegic migraine, which has been linked to a specific gene and is passed down from parent to child.

Migraine can also occur at any age. It's most common in people in their twenties and thirties, but children can suffer from migraine, as can the elderly. Although migraine is less common after the age of 50, it's far from rare. In fact, a study published in 1997 in the journal *Postgraduate Medicine* noted that migraine is the tenth most common complaint of elderly women and the fourteenth most common in elderly men.

There are racial differences as well. A study done in Baltimore County, reported in 1996 in the journal *Neurology*, found that although blacks and Asians suffer from migraines, they do so at a lower rate than Caucasians. This study found that Caucasian women had a migraine rate of 20.4 percent, compared to 16.2 percent for blacks and 9.2 percent for Asians. A similar pattern was observed in men, with 8.6 percent of Caucasians, 7.2 percent of blacks, and 4.2 percent of Asians reporting migraines. In addition, blacks were less likely to experience gastrointestinal symptoms, such as nausea or vomiting, but their head pain was more severe. The researchers concluded that these differences are most probably caused by genetic factors.

Many theories have been advanced to explain migraine. The first modern theory, which dates back to the 1600s, is known as the vascular theory, and in modified form it is still given weight today. According to this theory, a process called vasoconstriction causes the blood vessels in the occipital lobe of the brain to narrow, creating the visual disturbances known as aura. After this aura-causing spasm, a process called vasodilation occurs, in which the blood vessels widen. As a result, the nerves become irritated and inflamed, resulting in the painful throbbing of a migraine headache.

Another theory, known as the "serotonin theory," centers on the role played by the brain chemical serotonin. Serotonin, which serves a number of functions in the body, including the regulation of the blood vessels, is stored in the platelets of the blood and is released when these platelets clump together. Studies have shown that the platelets of migraineurs have a greater tendency to clump, which may release higher-than-normal amounts of serotonin, contributing to migraine. Serotonin has also been implicated in causing clinical depression and panic disorder, diseases which occur more often in migraineurs.

The "neurogenic theory" holds that migraine originates in the nerves, particularly those in the trigeminovascular system, which is the name given to a network of cranial nerves. According to this theory, the nerves become irritated and inflamed, releasing a chemical that causes pain messages to travel to the head and the face.

There's also the unifying theory, which seeks to combine aspects of all these theories. The contention here is that a migraine attack begins with electrical changes in the brain that affect the trigeminovascular system. These changes occur after a repeated onslaught of triggers an individual is sensitive to.

These triggers can vary from person to person. For some people, it may be alcohol, chocolate, or being exposed to certain chemicals or types of weather conditions. These known migraine triggers are discussed more fully later. For others, the triggers remain unknown. When the body can no longer take the stress these triggers cause, these electrical changes set off a cascade of biochemical events; the blood platelets clump, serotonin is released, and the blood vessels constrict. The result is inflammation and migraine pain.

There is still much we don't know about migraine. But the good news is that, nonetheless, there are more effective treatments to alleviate migraine now than ever before.

#7

LEARN WHAT CAUSES OTHER HEADACHES

Although it isn't known for sure what causes migraine, there are known causes for other types of headaches. Why is it essential that you learn about them? Because, as noted earlier, there's been a lot of confusion. People who think they get sinus headaches, for example, may actually be migraineurs. Or those who believe they get migraines may actually be experiencing severe tension headaches, for which the treatment may be different. Furthermore, it's not uncommon for migraineurs to suffer from other types of headache as well, and learning about them can help you get rid of this additional pain.

Here's a rundown on the causes of tension headache that can be mistakenly blamed for migraine.

Sinusitis: an inflammation of a sinus, or the sinuses, can result in a headache, as well as other symptoms such as nasal congestion, postnasal drip, mucus, face tenderness, or the sensation of an aching tooth.

Toothache: Often when you have a toothache, you can

readily identify the cause. Sometimes, though, this isn't the case. A toothache can manifest as a more generalized headache.

Eyestrain: If you find your headaches occur after doing close work, such as embroidery, or long stretches in front of a computer terminal or hunched over a textbook, the culprit may be eyestrain. A visit to the eye doctor is in order.

Temporomandibular (jaw) Disorder, known also as TMD or TMJ syndrome: This disorder has been blamed for a host of problems, including migraine, but most experts believe this problem has been blown way out of proportion.

TMD is a group of conditions, often painful, that affect the jaw joint and the muscles that control chewing. For most people, this jaw pain is not a signal of a serious problem. In fact, often it is temporary and occasional and goes away with little or no treatment, so only a small number of cases warrant corrective treatment. If you're told that you need expensive diagnostic tests or that you have TMD and require extensive, irreversible treatment, you'd be wise to get a second opinion. For a free booklet on TMD, see the Resources section.

Degenerative disorders: Certain diseases, such as rheumatoid arthritis and osteoporosis, which cause bones to become brittle, can affect the bones in the neck and result in headaches.

Posttraumatic headache: This is the name given to headaches that occur following a head injury or whiplash. Some people begin getting tension headaches, but those who develop migraines have symptoms that are identical to those suffered by other migraineurs. They usually respond to the same medications that relieve other forms of migraine.

Medication overuse: Medication, both prescription and over-the-counter, is a double-edged sword. On one hand, over-the-counter and prescription drugs can relieve headaches. On the other hand, although it's seldom recognized, these very same drugs can cause rebound headaches—which result as painkillers wear off and can cause frequent headaches that are very stubborn to treat. Rebound headaches are discussed in Chapter 25.

PART TWO

FOR WOMEN ONLY

#8

LEARN HOW MIGRAINES AFFECT YOU

Although migraine afflicts three times more women than men, it is not usually considered a serious "woman's disease" and not accorded the same attention as other ailments such as breast cancer or heart disease. Yet for the millions of women who suffer from it, migraine exacts a tremendous physical and emotional toll.

Consider the facts: Women get migraines more often than men; in fact, as a woman, you are three times more likely to get migraines. Your migraines also may be more severe and last longer, and you're more likely to experience auras, vomiting, and nausea.

The impact of a devastating migraine attack is likely to be harsher on you as well. Studies have found that women with migraines are less able to function at work, jeopardizing their careers more often. As a wife and mother, there may be times when you're unable to care for your children, straining your relationship at home and eating away at your sense of self-esteem. Your husband or partner may fail to understand the severity of your migraine disease, leading to the break-up of relationships and even divorce.

Indeed, a 1995 survey underscored these concerns. Because of their migraines, many women reported they lacked control of their lives, they lacked confidence, and they felt embarrassed and ashamed. Their migraines interfered with their ability to make plans, forced them to miss school plays and other activities, and robbed them of time spent with their husbands and children.

Even when they weren't in pain, migraine still colored their lives. At work, they tailored their day to avoid stress or found themselves unable to think clearly. At home, they put off making plans, fearing that a migraine could strike. Repeatedly, they voiced frustration, hopelessness, and loneliness.

Despite this sad picture, studies have found that most women with migraines don't seek treatment, and up to 40 percent of those who do are misdiagnosed or unsuccessfully treated. Even today, women are too often told that their headaches are "all in their heads" or that they have somehow brought their migraines on themselves by being too nervous or being unable to handle stress.

The following chapters deal with some special concerns of female migraineurs.

#9

FIND OUT IF YOU HAVE MENSTRUAL MIGRAINES

Up until puberty, boys and girls experience similar rates of migraine. After puberty, though, the balance shifts, and far more women are affected. Some of this difference is because women are more likely to experience migraines in relation to their menstrual cycle. Because of this, women too often think that all migraines are hormonally related. They're not, and determining which category you fall into can be very useful.

Only about 14 percent of female migraineurs meet the strict criteria of having true menstrual migraines, which means they occur only during their period. A far greater number of women, up to 60 percent, experience *menstrual-related* migraines. This means they get migraines more often during their period but also during other times of the month as well. The remaining 26 percent don't experience any correlation with their cycle, so their migraines aren't related to their hormones at all.

Menstrual migraines are often severe, unremitting, and among the most difficult to prevent or treat. Even worse, women who get these hormonally influenced migraines are often afflicted with regular migraines during the rest of the month.

Exactly what causes menstrual migraines isn't completely understood, but, as with other types of migraine, they run in families. The onset of menstrual migraines appears to be caused by fluctuations in a woman's hormones, particularly the hormone estrogen, which is believed to play a role in causing migraine.

Estrogen begins to rise toward the end of the menstrual flow of a woman's period. The amount of the hormone increases when ovulation occurs, around the fourteenth day, and remains high as the cycle draws to an end. If the egg is not fertilized, the levels of estrogen and progesterone will drop off around the twenty-fifth day and the lining of the uterus, which has been prepared to accept a fertilized egg, sloughs off, resulting in the start of the menstrual flow at day twenty-eight. The falling level of these hormones is what, in some women, triggers premenstrual mood changes, back pain, breast tenderness and headaches. And women who are prone to them get menstrual migraines.

Premenstrual migraines tend to occur right before the menstrual cycle and are relieved by the beginning of the flow, so sufferers are symptom-free between menstruation and ovulation. Menstrual migraines tend to cluster around the onset of menstruation, peaking on the first two days of bleeding. Women whose migraines are more loosely hormonally related may find their headaches occur at other times during the cycle, or mid-way, during ovulation.

The good news about menstrual and menstrual-related migraines is that there are effective treatments. Treatment regimens vary, but they encompass all the therapies discussed in this book for migraines in general, plus some additional ones utilizing hormones.

Although hormonal treatments may be very effective in women who get menstrual migraines, they may be useless in women who don't. That's why it's very important to keep a migraine calendar. Migraine calendars, explained later in the book (Chapter 37), are necessary to determine whether hormones play a role in your migraines. They can also rule out the influence of hormones; in fact, many women who assumed they get menstrual migraines learn, with the help of such a record, that they don't.

Knowing when you are vulnerable to menstrual migraines can help you make adjustments in your lifestyle that may help prevent them, notes Dr. Elizabeth Loder, director of the headache management program at Spaulding Rehabilitation Hospital in Boston.

"Women who get menstrual migraines find that their headache threshold is lowered [when the flow starts], meaning it's much easier for them to get a migraine. That doesn't mean it has to happen. There are things you can do to make it less likely to happen. You can be extra careful around that time of the month to eat right, stay away from your triggers, and get enough sleep," she says.

Chapter 37 tells how to keep a migraine calendar.

You should keep such a calendar for at least three months to establish the pattern of your headaches.

This calendar should include:

- Your age when you began menstruating
- The relationship of your migraines to your menstrual cycle and when you ovulate
- Any previous or current use of oral contraceptives
- Any changes in the menstrual flow
- If you're approaching or past menopause, any usage of postmenopausal replacement hormones

If you get severe menstrual migraines, you may need to turn to drugs for relief. Both abortive drugs, used to stop an attack, and preventative drugs, used to lessen the frequency or severity of migraines, can help. In addition, particularly for menstrual migraine, hormonal treatments that manipulate the body's level of estrogen can be very useful. These are used to smooth out the hormonal fluctuations believed to cause menstrual migraines. Your doctor may want to involve your gynecologist in your treatment plan as well.

DRUGS FOR MENSTRUAL MIGRAINE

Here's a brief rundown on some of the drugs used to treat menstrual migraines. To learn more about these drugs, and for important information on side effects, see Part IV: Using Drugs to Manage Migraine.

NSAIDS
Nonsteroidal antiinflammatory drugs, including naproxen sodium (Anaprox), fenoprofen calcium (Nalfon), naproxen (Naprosyn), ketoprofen (Orudis), and nabumetone (Relafen), have been found to be effective, especially when taken a few days before the start of the period and continued through the flow. For example, Dr. Fred Sheftell outlines, in his book *Headache Disorders*, a regimen for women whose migraines begin the first day of their menstrual flow. He has these women take naproxen sodium (either the prescription Anaprox or the over-the-counter drug Aleve), from four days before the estimated headache day to the end of their periods. He finds that this procedure relieves or lessens the pain for 30 to 50 percent of those who try it.

Ergotamine Tartrate
Ergotamine tartrate, combined in pill form with caffeine to enhance its effectiveness, should be taken as early as possible during an attack to be effective. It's available as oral tablets or, in the case of nausea, as a rectal suppository.

Dihydroergotamine Mesylate (D.H.E. 45)
An intravenous form of ergotamine, this drug is used at the first
sign of headache. It is available in a nasal spray, Migranal; by injection, or intravenously when given in an emergency room.

Isometheptene Mucate (Midrin)
This drug also helps relieve nausea and vomiting that may accompany migraines.

Sumatriptan (Imitrex)
Discussed at length later in the book, this drug is an effective
reliever of acute migraine. Studies have also found that it
relieves menstrual migraines and possibly cluster headaches
as well.

Hormonal Treatments
All the drugs just described are used in conventional migraine
treatment. Another way to prevent menstrual migraines is to
use an estrogen gel or patch or to give low-dose estrogen to
make sure one's estrogen level doesn't dip, triggering a migraine. Other hormonally based treatments include the anti-
estrogen drug tamoxifen (Nolvadex), or danazol (Danocrine),
which is a male hormone compound. These are strong drugs,
though, with possible side effects that include menopausal
symptoms.

   Although menstrual migraines can be difficult to treat, the
vast majority of women can find relief. To recap, here are
some tips:

- Use your migraine calendar to learn when you're most
  vulnerable.
- During this time, do all you can to avoid triggering a migraine. Steer clear of foods you're sensitive to, keep a
  regular schedule, and get enough rest.

- Take advantage of both the drug and nondrug therapies described later in this book that you find useful.
- Use your migraine calendar to keep track of what works—and doesn't work—for you. This can provide you with the incentive to make health choices during "that time of the month" and the rest of the time as well.

#10

Decide Whether to Take "The Pill"

Oral contraceptives, commonly known as birth control pills, are drugs used to prevent ovulation and, therefore, pregnancy. They may contain estrogen, or a combination of estrogen and progesterone, hormones that can influence the occurrence of migraine.

Since the introduction of the birth control pill over twenty-five years ago, there's been concern about migraine sufferers taking it. First and foremost, the pill was found to cause migraines in women who didn't otherwise get them, so it seemed obvious that women who did suffer from migraines should avoid the pill as well. Over the years, though, the pill has been reformulated, and the amount of hormones it contains has been reduced. As a result, the concern about migraine has lessened.

As with most aspects of migraine, the situation is not simple. In some women, the pill will bring on migraines. This has occasionally occurred even in women who don't have a family history of migraine. In some migraineurs, the pill will make their migraines worse. But some women find that the pill makes no difference at all and, even more perplexing, some women find that the pill actually improves their migraines. Some studies have found this to be the case most usually in women who have true menstrual migraines. There are no easy answers.

To understand how oral contraceptives impact migraine, you need to understand how they work. Oral contraceptives not only prevent pregnancy but they also work to mimic a woman's natural menstrual cycle. During this cycle, the amount of hormones in the blood fluctuates. To simulate this, a woman takes contraceptive pills containing hormones for 21 days. Then, she takes a placebo, which is a pill containing no active ingredients, for seven days. It is during this pill-free week that many women experience migraines.

There are two methods to reduce the possibility of migraine, suggests Dr. Merle Diamond, of the Diamond Headache Clinic. One method is to take a low dose of estrogen during the pill-free week. This keeps the hormone level stable, avoiding the dip that causes migraines. Another way to keep the hormone level stable is to use an estrogen patch to release estrogen slowly into the body. Either method may result in an occasional skipped period, but this should not cause any health problems, Dr. Diamond says.

But, as a migraineur, you also have to consider the possible connection between oral contraceptives and stroke. A review article published in 1997 in the *Canadian Journal of Neurological Sciences* discusses this issue.

You also have to consider that in the past, oral contraceptives were found to increase the risk of stroke. It's difficult to evaluate the research that's been done because over the years the formulas have changed, and the amount of estrogen the pill contains has been reduced. The overall risk of stroke in young women is low, but there is an increased risk for female migraineurs who take the pill, particularly those who experience prolonged auras or multiple neurological symptoms. The risk climbs if a woman smokes or has other stroke risk factors, including high blood pressure, heart disease, or a previous history of blood clots. These factors must all be considered when contemplating the use of oral contraceptives.

The 1997 article published in the *Canadian Journal of Neurological Sciences* states that those female migraineurs who don't fall into these categories can probably use oral contraceptives safely, but they should be reevaluated if their migraines significantly worsen or they start getting neurological symptoms, like weakness or numbness, confusion, dizziness, or difficulty speaking. Having migraine with aura doesn't necessarily rule out taking oral contraceptives; if you only experience fleeting neurological symptoms, your doctor may still think it's safe for you to use the pill, particularly a low-dose version. (For more information on stroke and migraine, see Chapter 19.)

In terms of treatment, women who continue to get migraines while on the pill generally respond to the same treatments used for menstrual migraines, which are described in the previous chapter.

So, if you are a migraineur, you should ask yourself these questions when considering oral contraceptives:

- Are there any preferable ways to prevent unwanted pregnancy?
- Are there medical reasons why I should be on the pill, such as to regulate menstrual irregularities?
- Do I have risk factors for stroke?

If you get menstrual migraines, oral contraceptives may or may not be the ideal contraceptive for you. Individuals vary, both in their risk factors and their response to the pill. But using this information can help you make the best decision.

#11

CONSIDER HOW MIGRAINE AFFECTS PREGNANCY

When Terri first became pregnant, she was thrilled. But she soon started worrying about how her pregnancy might affect her migraines. "I couldn't imagine having intense pain and constant vomiting while I was pregnant. I was also afraid of what effect taking my medication might have on the baby," Terri recalled.

Now, seven and a half months later, a clearly delighted, very pregnant Terri finds she need not have worried. "My migraines have disappeared!" she crows.

This isn't surprising. The temporary disappearance of migraine is often, although not always, a happy side effect of pregnancy.

WHICH PREGNANT WOMEN GET MIGRAINES?

As noted, the vast majority of women—some studies put it at 60 to 70 percent—experience relief from their migraines during pregnancy, especially the later months. In some women, though, migraine may appear for the first time during pregnancy. Some find their migraines worsen; still others experience no change. There is no way to predict which group you'll fall into, although some studies have shown that migraineurs experience relief more often than tension headache sufferers. Unfortunately, this blissful migraine-free period is usually temporary. Most of these women find their migraines return following childbirth, sometimes during breast-feeding, or after weaning. And that first returning migraine can be very severe! Although it's not fully understood why this occurs these changes in the migraine situation are apparently due to the hormonal fluctuations that occur in a woman's body during pregnancy and lactation.

MIGRAINES AND PREGNANCY

For pregnant women who continue to get migraines, or experience them for the first time, pregnancy raises some difficult issues.

The first involves diagnosis. If you're a known migraine sufferer, you generally won't need any further tests. But if you're a first-time migraine sufferer, or if you're experiencing changes in your headaches, your doctor may want to do further evaluation. This is especially true in the following scenarios.

- You experience a sudden, severe headache, such as the type called a thunderclap headache, which comes on suddenly and reaches maximum intensity within one minute.
- Your migraines have become more frequent or more severe.
- You've begun experiencing auras for the first time or you have neurological symptoms that linger or occur without headache.

- You experience severe head pain with exertion.
- You faint or experience seizures.

If your doctor does recommend diagnostic testing, and you know or think you may be pregnant, speak up, so the doctor can choose tests that will not present an unnecessary risk to your unborn child.

TREATING MIGRAINES DURING PREGNANCY

The most common and most difficult issue that arises during pregnancy is what medications to prescribe when migraines occur. It's essential for a woman's peace of mind to know that she doesn't have to choose between enduring agonizing pain and delivering a healthy baby, but too often this has been the case, says Dr. Elizabeth Loder, who has written extensively on the subject. "The management strategy I often see is 'Let's wait as long as we can and then do as little as possible, and see if we can manage until the end of the pregnancy,' " she states.

Doctors have taken an extremely cautious approach toward giving drugs to pregnant women since the early 1960s, when the drug thalidomide was discovered to cause birth defects. Although the drug was never approved in this country, its impact was so devastating that doctors began to take a dim view of pregnant women taking drugs, a viewpoint that continues to this day. The thalidomide tragedy also caused the FDA to prohibit the testing of drugs in pregnant women. This effectively banned the testing of drugs in women in general, as even non-pregnant women were seen as those who could become so. The FDA recently reversed this policy, but gathering data to close the gap will take years. Therefore, many doctors avoid giving drugs to pregnant women because their potential side effects are not known.

In his article "Migraine and Pregnancy," published in 1997 in the journal *Neurologic Clinics*, Stephen D. Silberstein, M.D., of the Comprehensive Headache Center at Germantown Hospital and Medical Center in Philadelphia, explores this subject in depth.

Despite the cautions, pregnant women continue to take drugs, writes Dr. Silberstein, and he cites several studies to back up his claim. He also contends that some drugs are safe for pregnant women to use, but this doesn't mean they should be widely recommended, since many drugs do have the potential to injure the fetus. Therefore, medication should be used as judiciously as possible. However, he adds, drugs may be necessary for women who continue to have "severe, intractable headaches, sometimes associated with nausea, vomiting and possible dehydration." These migraines not only are distressing for the sufferers but also may pose a risk to the fetus "that is greater than the potential risk of the medications used to treat the pregnant patient," he writes.

There are two major classifications of drugs given to migraineurs: first, "abortive" drugs, taken at the time of the attack to relieve it; second, "preventative" drugs, which can reduce the frequency and severity of migraine. These are discussed in general later in this book.

Many abortive drugs can be hazardous during pregnancy and should not be taken. Some, however, such as Tylenol and some types of NSAIDs, may be used. You must discuss these first with your doctor, because some may be safe during some stages of pregnancy but not in others. Narcotics carry the potential of addiction for both mother and baby. Ergotamine and ergotamine derivatives, useful for menstrual migraines, can harm the developing fetus. Newer drugs, such as sumatriptan (Imitrex), are not yet approved for pregnant women.

Preventative drugs generally are not considered safe for pregnant women although, again, this is a topic you need to discuss with your doctor.

Bear in mind, though, that all drugs are not unsafe. If you suffer from severe attacks, and your doctor bans the use of drugs, you might want to seek a second opinion from a migraine specialist.

To recap, here are some things to remember if you are pregnant or planning to become so:

- Talk to your doctor immediately. Generally, your doctor will want to discontinue any preventative migraine medication you're taking as far in advance of becoming pregnant as possible, and carefully monitor the abortive medications you take as well.
- Your doctor may advise you to get pregnant as quickly as possible, so you can minimize the time of uncertainty when you don't know whether you should take medication because you don't know if you're pregnant.
- Remember, if you are contemplating pregnancy, this may turn into a migraine-free period. But even if it doesn't, there are ways to make this period as pain-free and blissful as it should be.

#12

DECIDE ABOUT HORMONE REPLACEMENT THERAPY

"It's really been miraculous," noted Carole, a fifty-one-year-old artist. "All of my life, it seems, I got migraines. But ever since I passed menopause, they seem to have vanished. Everyone told me what a problem menopause could be, with hot flashes and all, but this is about the best thing that ever happened to me," she exclaimed.

Menopause, the time which signals the end of your reproductive cycles, along with other biological passages in a woman's life, is a time of great hormonal changes. If your migraines are affected by hormones, menopause may have a great impact on your migraines as well, and that change may be welcome. Often, women who suffer from menstrual migraines report that, following menopause, their migraines disappear. But, as you'll see, this isn't true for everyone. Also, menopause brings with it special issues.

The average age when a woman reaches menopause is fifty-one, but some women become menopausal as early as in their forties or as late as their sixties.

Menopause seems to have a variable effect on migraine. Studies find that some women report their migraines improve, or disappear, after menopause. However, a minority of women report their migraines begin as they near menopause, during the time known as "perimenopause" and others report no change.

Menopause used to be considered as a specific time in a woman's life. Now, though, it's known that these hormonal changes that culminate in menopause begin slowly, and can stretch over months, or even more than a year. This is known as "perimenopause."

During perimenopause, the ovaries become less capable of producing estrogen and progesterone. Because the ovaries can no longer produce estrogen, the pituitary gland, recognizing there is a low estrogen level in the blood stream, sends out signals to make more estrogen, resulting in hormone fluctuations. It is during perimenopause that some women report their migraines worsen. But upon entering menopause, usually viewed as the year following a woman's final period, many menstrual migraine sufferers report their attacks have at last disappeared.

WHAT ABOUT HORMONE REPLACEMENT THERAPY?

Many postmenopausal women take hormone replacement therapy, natural or synthetic hormones designed to counteract the symptoms of menopause, on a short-term basis to eliminate such problems as hot flashes and night sweats. But lately there has been a trend to prescribe these hormones on a long-term basis, possibly forever, to women in hopes of their warding off osteoporosis, heart disease, and possibly other maladies of aging, including Alzheimer's disease.

The long-term use of hormone replacement therapy brings with it implications that all women should consider. Although the long-term hormones have been found to definitely or possibly reduce the risk of the above-mentioned diseases, they also increase the risk of breast cancer.

But, if you get menstrual migraines, there's another issue you must weigh as well. Because taking hormone replacement therapy is designed to replicate the female menstrual cycle, they replicate the very conditions that result in menstrual migraines. This is an unwelcome side effect for the woman who has suffered from these migraines for years, only to find relief after going through menopause.

Few studies have been done on the effect of hormone replacement therapy on migraines and the ones that have been done report varying results. In some cases, women report that their migraines improve, others say they worsen, and still others report no change.

In any case, there are ways to manipulate replacement hormones to minimize this problem. Most migraineurs who take hormone replacement therapy find they suffer their attacks when they take the hormones according to the schedule most commonly given. This regimen calls for a woman to take estrogen for twenty-one days, followed by seven days in which it is not taken. Progesterone is usually given for ten days of the month. Women often report they feel worse during the days they take no estrogen, and still worse on the days they take progesterone.

However, administering postmenstrual hormones continuously, so the amount in the body remains stable, by using an estrogen patch or estrogen pills, can help cut the rate of postmenopausal migraine by 50 percent.

In making your decision, consider not only your migraines, but also your overall medical reason for wishing to take hormones. You can take them on a trial basis and taper off if they make your migraines worse. Don't stop taking them suddenly, though, or you can experience a return of menopausal symptoms. If the hormones do worsen your migraines, but you want to continue taking them, discuss the issue with your doctor. You may need to enlist the help of both a gynecologist and a headache specialist working together to find a regimen that works for you.

PART THREE

GET
PROFESSIONAL
HELP

#13

CHOOSE THE RIGHT DOCTOR

This is a self-help book, packed with treatments you can try and lifestyle changes you can make yourself. But since migraine is a biological disease, it makes sense that you may need medical help. Some migraine sufferers are able to find relief on their own. But you should consider seeking a doctor's help if:

- You suffer from frequent or severe migraines
- You have never discussed your migraines with a doctor
- Your symptoms have changed or worsened
- You are using over-the-counter headache medications frequently and still getting headaches or migraines

Unfortunately, seeking help can be frustrating. This was especially true in the past, when little could be done to help, and migraine sufferers were viewed as complainers. This view is changing, but you may still encounter it, especially if you're a woman, notes Dr. Grace Steere, an internist who herself is a migraine sufferer.

"Because the pain is so tremendous and a lot of doctors have the attitude, 'Oh, it's another female with headaches,' migraine sufferers tend to get brushed aside," she says.

It's not surprising, therefore, that many sufferers delay seeking help. In fact, a 1994 survey of two hundred doctors found that people with migraine suffered for an average of three and a half years before seeking treatment. The same survey found that, even when they did seek help, patients couldn't accurately convey their degree of pain, symptoms, or medical history—essential elements in getting the right diagnosis and treatment.

When it comes to selecting a doctor to treat migraines, there are essential decisions to make.

First, you must decide which type of doctor to see. Unfortunately, there's no simple answer to that question. It seems logical that, since migraine is a neurological disease, a neurologist, who deals with diseases of the brain, would be the ideal choice. Sometimes that's true, especially if the doctor is particularly interested in the treatment of migraine. But general practitioners, internists, or primary care physicians can also provide good care.

In the past, migraine patients had a reputation for being difficult. In part, that's due to all the myths that surround this disease. So if you suspect that a doctor may automatically be prejudiced against you because you get migraines, you may not be imagining the reaction. Furthermore, since migraine is a problem of chronic pain, which is notoriously difficult to treat, many doctors prefer not to deal with migraine patients at all.

Unfair? Yes. An impossible problem to overcome? No. If you select your doctor carefully, you'll find that many caring practitioners exist.

How can you tell if your doctor is the right one for you? There are no guarantees but sometimes, there are tipoffs.

It's a positive sign if your doctor has published articles about migraine, but this is a very specialized area, and relatively few do. Organizations listed in the Resources section, such as the American Council of Headache Education (ACHE), the National Headache Foundation, or Migraine Awareness Group: A National Understanding For Migraineurs (M.A.G.N.U.M.), can refer you to doctors who specialize in migraine. But don't rule out a doctor who isn't formally involved in the field. Some doctors who don't specialize in headaches can be knowledgeable and sensitive, just as some specialists may not be the right doctor for you.

Choose your doctor carefully. After all, migraine is a complex disease, and you and your doctor need to forge a long-standing relationship. Question your doctor about the causes and treatment for migraine. If you receive answers that are outdated, choose someone else. Pay attention to the manner in which your doctor answers these questions. If your doctor seems curt or uninterested, this is an indication that you should consider choosing someone else. Your doctor should also be willing to give you a procedure to use in case your migraines become so severe that you need emergency help.

Remember, though, that migraine treatment is not a one-way street. The success in managing migraines depends a lot on you. Ask yourself honestly:

- Am I willing to tell my doctor about all the medications I am taking?
- Am I willing to give medications a fair trial?
- Am I willing to treat my doctor with the same respect that I expect?

Migraine is a frustrating and challenging problem. A good, communicative relationship between you and your doctor can be the cornerstone to getting the best help.

#14

KNOW YOUR MEDICAL HISTORY

To make the most of your doctor's appointment, you should bring along your medical history—written down. This is more essential than ever as, due to changes in the health care industry, doctors' visits are getting shorter and shorter. Your medical history provides information needed to help your doctor more accurately diagnose and treat your migraine problem. Your medical history also provides important clues about which drugs to prescribe and what lifestyle changes might be helpful, and it can open the door to other vital areas of discussion.

To create your medical history, first make sure you answered the ten questions at the beginning of this book (see Chapter 4). Now here are some more questions. Answer them in writing, even if you're not planning to see a doctor. The answers can help you map your own treatment plan.

- Do you have, or do you have a family history of, the following medical conditions?
  — Neurological problems, epilepsy, or seizures

- — High blood pressure
- — Abnormal cholesterol
- — Chest pain/angina
- — Heart attack
- — Heart disease or Raynaud's disease
- — Diabetes
- Have you experienced any accidents or blows to the head?
- Have you been diagnosed with depression or panic disorder, or have you ever attempted suicide?
- Are you taking any of the following medications?
  - — High blood pressure drugs
  - — Headache or migraine drugs
  - — Over-the-counter drugs (for migraine or any other conditions)
- Include this information if you are female:
  - — Whether your headaches began when you began menstruating
  - — If and when the headaches occur during your monthly menstrual cycle
  - — Whether you're approaching, going through, or past menopause
  - — Whether you are pregnant or plan to be pregnant soon
  - — Your headache history during pregnancy and after giving birth and/or nursing
  - — Whether you're taking oral contraceptives
  - — Whether you're on hormone replacement therapy

Your doctor's medical history form may be even more detailed than this list. In any event, providing accurate answers to these questions can form the basis of an effective treatment plan.

#15

LEARN THE FACTS ABOUT DIAGNOSTIC TESTS

For migraine sufferers, diagnostic tests can be frustrating. It's only human nature to long for a definitive test that will prove, once and for all, that you are suffering from migraine. What most sufferers eventually end up with, though, is a thick file of tests results that read "normal." Sometimes the migraineur, beset with frustration and fear from the attacks, will insist on more tests, and the cycle will begin anew.

This scenario is all too frequent. There are indeed certain cases in which diagnostic testing is warranted. But for many migraine sufferers, all the testing that's available may not furnish any useful information.

As yet there is no definitive test that can "prove" whether or not you suffer from migraines. So the diagnosis of migraine is one of elimination—the elimination of other potential causes of head pain. Adding to the confusion is the fact that doctors differ on what they believe constitutes necessary testing. Your doctor may simply take a medical history, but your friend's doctor may subject her to a battery of sophisticated medical imaging tests. Neither is necessarily right or wrong; there's just no uniformly accepted regimen of testing.

Generally, though, if you are seeing your doctor for the first time about migraines, your doctor will want to rule out other potentially serious causes of headache. This is especially true if:

- Your symptoms don't conform to those of a typical migraine
- You've only just begun getting headaches
- Your headaches have become worse or more frequent
- You've only just begun experiencing auras or other neurological symptoms
- You have any of the warning signs described in the next chapter

THE TESTS

Here are some of the tests that you may encounter.

Physical Exam

A physical exam is the diagnostic test most commonly done, and it should be performed especially if you're asking a doctor about your migraines for the first time. This exam is done to rule out any conditions that can be mistaken for migraine or to uncover any warning signs that warrant further investigation. Such an exam includes checking your vital signs, including your blood pressure, to make sure it isn't high, and your temperature, to make sure you don't have an infection. The doctor will also check to make sure you have a full range of motion in your neck, to rule out meningitis.

Blood Chemistry Test

This test is done to make sure you don't have anemia or any other more serious blood disease. Blood chemistry tests can rule out disorders such as hepatitis or renal dysfunction. If you live in an area where Lyme disease is common, it should also be ruled out.

Many doctors will call a halt to testing at this point, if all indications point to migraine and the patient is otherwise healthy. But there are some other tests you may encounter, as follows.

Electroencephalography (EEG)

In this test, a number of small electrodes are placed on the scalp and connected to an instrument that measures and records the electrical impulses produced by the brain. This testing in migraineurs is controversial because, although irregularities may be found, there is disagreement over whether they are significant or not. But this test should be performed if there is a history of seizures, loss of consciousness, head trauma, or sudden dizzy spells.

Computed Axial Tomography (CT or CAT scan)

This is a sophisticated imaging test that uses a computer that merges many X rays from several angles into a single picture. It can be performed with or without a contrasting dye. This test can diagnose ailments such as brain tumors and blood clots— rare problems indeed, but ones that do cause headache.

Magnetic Resonance Imaging (MRI)

Like the CT scan, the MRI is a sophisticated diagnostic device. The machine uses a strong magnet to obtain thousands of views of the brain, which a computer then blends into one accurate image. Unlike a CT scan, an MRI can differentiate between normal and abnormal tissues, so it can detect problems at an early stage.

Once liberally used on headache patients, CT scans and MRIs are now usually reserved for cases in which abnormalities are suspected. According to practice guidelines issued by the Quality Standards Subcommittee of the American Academy of

Neurology, CT scans and MRIs should not be used in adults whose headaches fit within the broad definition of migraine unless they have experienced a substantial change in their headache pattern—such as seizures or abnormal neurological signs—or they have developed a headache after a blow or other trauma to the head.

Migraineurs often believe these sophisticated testing devices can detect more than is actually possible. According to a study published in 1994 in the *Canadian Medical Association Journal*, very few abnormalities were found in people with severe, chronic headaches who underwent CT scans. In fact, this study found that when the same number of people without headaches were tested, the same number of abnormalities were found.

Certainly, if you've already had such tests, tell your doctor, so that copies can be obtained, saving time and money. If your doctor is dissatisfied with the quality of those tests, they can be redone.

If your doctor pays careful attention to your symptoms but doesn't order extensive tests, don't be dismayed. Often patients, and their doctors, overestimate the usefulness of tests in diagnosing migraines, and patients end up being overtested.

Usually the most telling test is the passage of time. If you get attacks interspersed with periods of time in which you feel fine, then this is a test in itself that can demonstrate that you're suffering from migraine.

#16

CONSIDER A HEADACHE CLINIC

In many cases, migraines can be treated by doctors who are considered nonspecialists, such as primary care physicians and internists. Indeed, in these days of managed care, this is the doctor you're most likely to see. Or you may be seen by a neurologist or other type of specialist. However, if you have a severe migraine or complicated headache problem, you may require the resources of a headache clinic.

The first specialized headache clinic was founded in 1945 at Montefiore Hospital in the Bronx, New York. Since then, many more have sprung up across the country. At a headache clinic, you're seen by not only a doctor but also a team that can address problems as needed. This team can include a psychologist, nutritionist, relaxation specialist, and others. You'll be given whatever diagnostic tests are deemed appropriate and, at the end of the evaluation, receive a migraine management plan.

An important benefit of headache clinics is that the doctors and all the staff are trained to be sensitive to the needs of the migraineur. Such sensitivity is sometimes, but not always, found in other settings.

Obviously, doctors not affiliated with headache specialists can offer some of these services, but it's not cost-effective for most to do so. At headache treatment centers, headaches are the only area of concern.

At a 1996 conference for headache professionals in Florida, Frederick G. Freitag, D.O., associate director of the Diamond Headache Clinic in Chicago, outlined some reasons for seeking help from such a clinic:

- Your doctor cannot arrive at a diagnosis of your headache type, or you suffer from "mixed headache syndrome." This means you may not only have migraine but another type of headache as well.
- You may be unable to tolerate the necessary drugs or other therapy for your migraines, or you may have built up a tolerance for the conventional treatments.
- You may have another medical condition that could interfere with your migraine treatment (or vice versa), such as high blood pressure, asthma, or diabetes.
- You've become dependent on certain types of drugs, or you've developed rebound headaches from overusing them.
- Your migraines have resulted in psychological or psychiatric problems.

Most headache clinics are run on an outpatient basis; there are a few inpatient ones. Costly inpatient care is generally reserved for patients who are seriously addicted to pain medication, suffer unrelenting, prolonged pain that has been impossible to relieve by other means, or have other unusually severe problems.

If you think a headache clinic will benefit you, discuss the possibility with your doctor. There's a hitch, though. As managed care and other cost-conscious health insurance plans become more common, referrals to such clinics are becoming increasingly difficult to obtain. As a result, "by the time people get here, they are much sicker, they are taking more addicting medication, they have developed more side effects," said Dr. Fred Sheftell, director of the New England Center for Headache in Stamford, Connecticut.

If you belong to a managed health care plan, you may need to assert yourself. See Chapter 49 for more on how to make sure you get the medical coverage you're entitled to.

#17

TREAT DEPRESSION, PANIC DISORDER

What are the subjects of depression and panic disorder doing in a book about migraines?

Too often in the past, migraine sufferers were told that their problem stemmed from "nerves" or "depression." But, just as it's been found that migraine is a medical disease, not a psychological one, it's becoming clearer that depression and panic disorder are biologically based as well. And studies find that people who get migraines are more likely to suffer from one, the other, or even both.

Obviously, someone who suffers from migraine attacks has very good reason to be depressed. But several studies demonstrate a link between clinical depression and migraine. For example, research on 1,007 adults reported in 1995 in the journal *Headache* found that the risk of developing depression was more than three times higher for persons with migraine. An earlier study, published in 1992 in the journal *Cephalalgia*, looked at a random sampling of 995 young adults and found that those with migraine were four times more likely to be depressed, whether they had suffered any recent migraine attacks or not.

Although the research which links panic disorder with migraine is not as voluminous as the studies on migraine and depression, there does appear to be a link. In 1994 research published in the journal *Neurology,* more than ten thousand people with panic disorder were asked if they had headaches. Of the four types of headaches defined, only migraine was found to have a strong link. Also, the study mentioned earlier in the journal *Cephalalgia,* which looked at the connection between migraine and depression, found that people with a history of migraine were twelve times as likely to develop panic disorder.

What is the connection between these diseases? Researchers aren't sure, but they speculate that these three problems may share the same underlying biological cause, possible abnormalities in the working of the brain chemical serotonin.

If you get treatment for migraines, but ignore these other ailments, your attempts to find relief may fail. As the authors of a 1997 paper published in the journal *Neurologic Clinics* note, when depression or panic disorder are also present, "it is critical to treat the entire syndrome," and not just limit treatment to migraine.

DEPRESSION

Clinical depression is more than just "feeling blue," or being depressed due to an obvious reason, such as having severe migraines.

How do you know you're clinically depressed? Here are the warning signs of depression. If they describe how you feel, discuss them with your doctor:

- Negativity in all aspects of life. This includes feelings of pessimism, hopelessness, worthlessness, and believing that nothing can make your life better.
- Sleep disturbances. Sleeping problems typically include being unable to fall asleep, waking in the middle of the night and being unable to go back to sleep, and sleeping too much.
- Appetite disturbances, such as eating too much or lacking an appetite, gaining or losing weight.
- Feelings of fatigue or a lack of energy that permeates everything you do.
- Loss of interest in usual activities, including work, activities you usually enjoyed, and sex.
- Trouble concentrating or making decisions.
- Persistent sadness or bouts of crying.
- Suicidal thoughts.

If you suffer from clinical depression, this can affect your migraine treatment. For example, beta blockers are often used as a migraine preventative, but they can cause depression. On the other hand, Prozac (fluoxetine), an antidepressant, is also a migraine preventative and may be a better choice for someone who is depressed. But, when used for migraines, the dosage is usually less, so care must be taken so the proper amount is prescribed to alleviate both problems.

Also, too often, people who are depressed discover that taking certain migraine abortive drugs, such as those containing narcotics or barbiturates, can temporarily lift their depression. As a result, they may misuse their drugs and possibly become addicted (this is true for people who suffer from panic disorder as well).

Depression also results in a sense of hopelessness that can make a migraine problem seem worse or sap your resolve to take steps that could help alleviate it.

PANIC DISORDER

We all worry about things, but when does normal worrying turn into the problem known as panic disorder?

Panic disorder consists of excessive, prolonged, almost daily anxiety and worry about a variety of activities or events. In addition, the person experiences three or more of the following symptoms:

- Restlessness
- Easy fatigue
- Difficulty concentrating
- Irritability
- Tense muscles
- Disturbed sleep

People with panic disorder can experience panic attacks, sudden, powerful feelings of dread, apprehension, and a sense of impending doom. This is often accompanied by heart palpitations, shortness of breath, weakness, sweating, choking, nausea, and numbness or tingling in the hands and feet. These symptoms can be so severe you may think you're having a heart attack. Since sufferers usually link their attack to a specific place where it occurred, like an elevator, airplane, or crowded store, eventually they begin avoiding these places, and their activities can become narrowed. Women, particularly, can become afraid to leave their homes, a disorder known as agoraphobia.

As with depression, people who suffer from anxiety and migraines may end up misusing drugs such as barbiturates or narcotics in a futile attempt to treat their anxiety. Too often, the result is that neither problem is alleviated.

Panic disorder is frightening, but the good news is that it is treatable. Treatments include drugs, including Prozac. Another effective treatment is a type of therapy known as cognitive-behavioral therapy, in which the person's thought patterns are retrained, enabling them to put their fears into perspective. This is sometimes used alone or in combination with drug therapy.

Like migraine, depression and anxiety can be frustrating problems. But there are more effective ways to treat all three of these problems than ever before.

#18

LEARN THESE IMPORTANT WARNING SIGNS

Very often, migraine is described as a disorder that feels like it will kill you, even though it won't. Sometimes it's characterized this way to avoid unduly alarming migraineurs, who sometimes don't believe that their excruciating pain could be harmless. Nonetheless, severe head pain can be an important warning sign of a serious medical condition. Such problems include brain tumors, an impending stroke caused by a blood clot or hemorrhage in the brain, and a disease such as infectious meningitis or encephalitis.

Getting migraines also increases your risk of stroke. Strokes are rare in the young and middle-aged (the groups most likely to get migraine), but they do occur. Stroke in migraineurs is discussed in the next chapter.

Since the pain of migraine is so excruciating, it's not surprising that migraineurs can fear that they have a life-threatening medical condition. This is usually not the case. But you should be aware of the following warning signs. They don't always signal a dangerous situation, but they may signal a need for testing and treatment.

Here are the warning signs:

- You get head pain that starts suddenly, is constant, and progressively increases in intensity.
- Your head pain was precipitated by a blow or injury to the head.
- Your head pain is much more severe than it's been in the past.
- Your head pain prevents you from going about your normal activity to an unusual extent. People who get migraines often can't go about their usual activities, but this is meant to denote a migraine that is so extreme it doesn't fit your usual pattern.
- Your head pain is accompanied by any unusual neurological symptoms, such as a temporary loss or change of vision, motor abilities, or sensation. If these are the changes that normally accompany your headache, don't be alarmed. But if you ordinarily don't get auras, for example, and you start getting them, contact your doctor. It's common for migraineurs who experience auras to experience headaches without them, but it's less common for those who don't get auras to suddenly begin experiencing them.
- Your neck becomes stiff, you have a fever, or you experience night sweats, chills, loss of weight, loss of appetite, muscle pain, or other signs of illness.
- You're over forty, you've never suffered from migraines, and you begin getting them, or any type of headaches. It's quite possible for people to begin experiencing migraines when they're older, and it may not signify any additional medical problem. But since older people are more at risk for other medical conditions, you should be checked out.
- You suffer from occasional migraines, but they begin increasing in number or becoming worse.

- Your head pain worsens rapidly and reaches a crescendo within five minutes.
- Your head pain is accompanied by personality changes, seizures, weakness, excessive sleepiness, lethargy, or loss of consciousness.

Consult your doctor promptly if any of these warning signs occur.

#19

REDUCE YOUR RISK OF STROKE

Because migraine can temporarily cause slurred speech, numbness, and other symptoms similar to stroke, it's only natural to wonder if being a migraineur increases your risk of this leading cause of death and disability. It's also natural to wonder if a particularly severe migraine can cause a stroke.

These questions seem clearcut, but the answers are not. Study results are conflicting, but most indicate that getting migraine does increase your risk of a stroke, although there's disagreement about how much.

It's difficult to pin down the exact answer, because there are inconsistencies on how such strokes are classified. Numbers are also elusive because it's often difficult for the sufferer to distinguish between migraine attacks and early signs of stroke. Moreover, research has given conflicting results, with some studies finding no increase and others finding almost a fourfold increase. Generally, it's thought that the true number lies somewhere in between.

A true "migrainous stroke," which is a stroke that occurs

during a migraine, is one in which the neurological symptoms last at least several days or there is evidence of stroke on a CT scan or MRI, says Nabih M. Ramadan, M.D., director of the Cincinnati Headache Center, who specializes in this subject.

It isn't known how often such strokes occur, but it's generally thought that, if you get migraines, especially with aura, your risk of stroke is about double that of the general population. If you get migraines without aura, your risk is less, although it's still more than nonmigraineurs.

Statistically, this means that migraine may account for up to as many as ten thousand strokes a year in the eight million Americans who suffer from migraine with aura. Research also indicates the risk is higher for women under the age of thirty-five.

Furthermore, if you fall into this category, your risk of suffering a stroke is increased if you have other stroke risk factors, such as high blood pressure, or if you smoke or take birth control pills.

According to several studies, including one published in 1997 in the *Archives of Neurology*, this holds true for both men and women. This study, done at Yale University, analyzed data from twelve thousand people and found that migraine conferred risk even in the absence of other known stroke risk factors. This study also found that the risk of stroke diminished with age.

The exact reason why migraine increases stroke risk is not known. Dr. Ramadan believes it may be linked to the period during a migraine in which the blood flow is reduced to the brain. In the Yale research, the authors also speculated that it may have something to do with an abnormality in the cardiac or the immune systems.

Not everyone believes that migraine causes a significant number of strokes. Dr. Marie-Germaine Bousser, past president of the International Headache Society, contends that migraineurs shouldn't be alarmed, because the general risk of stroke is so low. She agrees, however, that some groups are at particular risk, especially young women who smoke and take birth control pills. She cited a study done at her own institution, the Hospital Saint-Antoine in Paris, in which the medical records of two hundred stroke victims were compared with an equal number of healthy participants. Female migraineurs who smoked and took oral contraceptives had triple the stroke risk, especially if they experienced auras, the study found.

What does this mean for you? Although it's not known exactly how much added risk migraine contributes, it plays a part. Therefore, you should do all you can to minimize your risk of stroke.

How do you know if you are at higher risk? Bear in mind that auras in typical migraine patients last about thirty minutes or less. So if you typically experience auras that last for more than an hour, you may be at higher risk. This is particularly true for those who suffer from hemiplegic auras or who experience any paralysis. If you do, you should take steps to minimize your risk factors for stroke, such as smoking and using birth control pills. Dr. Ramadan also suggests that you take care not to strain your neck by doing such vigorous activities as high jumping or diving, and that you avoid chiropractic neck manipulation.

Furthermore, he notes that sumatriptan, or any of the drugs now being developed that act similarly, shouldn't be used by this group of people because it may cause constriction of the cardiovascular system. These drugs are already contraindicated in people who get hemiplegic and basilar migraines, he noted.

To sum up, if you're a migraineur, your risk of stroke is higher than nonmigraineurs but is still low. However, you should be aware of these modifiable risk factors for stroke and do all you can to minimize them:

- High blood pressure
- Coronary heart disease
- Diabetes
- Smoking
- Smoking and taking oral contraceptives

If you are a female migraineur who smokes and takes birth control pills and you want to continue using oral contraceptives, you should make sure they contain the lowest amount of estrogen possible.

You should also be aware of the warning signs of stroke. Since some of these warning signs are identical to the symptoms that occur in a migraine attack with aura, it's often very difficult to tell them apart. However, if you experience neurological symptoms that are unusual for you, or if your aura lasts longer than usual, or if you experience paralysis, you should contact your doctor. The only exception would be if you get hemiplegic migraines in which paralysis is a common symptom or if this type of migraine runs in your family. In addition, if you're over forty and experiencing a migraine and/or aura symptoms for the first time, your doctor should evaluate you and not just assume you have a migraine.

Here, then, are the warning signs of stroke:

- Sudden weakness or numbness of the face, arm, or leg on one side of the body
- Sudden difficulty speaking or understanding others
- Dimness or impaired vision, particularly in only one eye or half of both eyes
- Sudden confusion
- Sudden unexplained dizziness
- Sudden onset of unsteadiness or lack of coordination, difficulty walking, or falling
- Sudden excruciating headache

- Recent change in personality or mental abilities, including memory loss

There is also a condition known as transient ischemic attacks (TIAs) or ministrokes. The symptoms of TIAs are the same as those of stroke, but they are only temporary. However, TIAs warn of impending strokes, so anyone experiencing them should seek medical help immediately.

Complicating the matter, though, is that there is a rare type of migraine variant known as aura without headache, which produces symptoms that can be confused with a stroke. Only your doctor can definitely determine which you are experiencing.

PART FOUR

Using Drugs to Manage Migraine

#20

LEARN THE FACTS ABOUT DRUGS

There's nothing Steve dreads more than a migraine. He began getting them when he was twelve. He used to despair of finding anything to help him. But he finally saw a doctor who gave him a drug that drastically shortens his attacks. Now he says, "I still hate to get migraines more than anything, but I know I can do something about it, so that lessens the anxiety."

Regarding drugs, there's lots to know about which to use and when to use them.

"When I first started working in the migraine field about twenty years ago, there was a handful of drugs we could use. Now there are literally hundreds," says Dr. R. Michael Gallagher, author of the book *Drug Therapy for Headache*. Over the years drugs have played an important role in the treatment of migraine, and this is becoming ever more true, especially with the development of many new drugs designed to treat only this disease. In order to find the most effective treatment for you, there is specific information you need to know.

Generally, drugs used to treat migraine fall into two categories: abortive and preventative. Most migraineurs need an abortive medication to use during acute attacks. Some migraineurs may also find it useful to take a preventative drug on a steady basis to reduce the number of migraines they get.

No matter what type of drugs you're using, remember these essentials:

1. Use the mildest medication possible to provide relief. More severe migraines warrant stronger pain medication.

2. Read and take seriously the warnings about drug rebound in Chapter 25.

3. Nondrug therapies, such as biofeedback and acupuncture, help many people. So do dietary changes, exercising, and other lifestyle measures. Employing a combination of all these methods may provide you with the most effective help.

Here are the guidelines doctors use when deciding which drugs to provide.

First, what type of headache do you have? Some medications work wonders for migraines but don't work at all if you are plagued with a combination of migraine and tension headache.

Second, doctors usually try milder medications first, reserving the more powerful for later on, if needed. Thus, your doctor will probably want to try an analgesic or mild blood vessel constrictor before turning to a narcotic or one of the more potent migraine relievers. Before you insist on the latest migraine drug, make sure that there aren't milder medications that will offer relief.

Third, your doctor will want to know about any medical conditions you have or other medications you're taking. "There are precautions with virtually every medication. The doctor has to be cautious based on the patient's medical history, other disease conditions, and so forth," notes Robert Rosum, a pharma-

cist who specializes in headache treatment at the New England
Center for Headache in Stamford, Connecticut.

Sometimes migraine can be treated with nonprescription
drugs. But more often, prescribing just the right combination of
drugs to relieve or prevent migraine, while weighing all the potential side effects, requires the skill of a practitioner who is up
to date on current migraine treatment. Form an alliance with
your local pharmacist as well; he or she can often be an excellent resource.

#21

LEARN ABOUT
ABORTIVE DRUGS

Americans spend approximately one billion dollars a year on nonprescription headache relievers. Nonprescription drugs are often the first line of defense against migraine. These drugs can be divided into four categories:

- Aspirin (this includes buffered and nonbuffered aspirin)
- Acetaminophen, such as Tylenol
- Nonsteroidal anti-inflammatory drugs (NSAIDs), such as ibuprofen (Advil, Mediprin, Motrin IB, Nuprin) or naproxen sodium, marketed as Aleve
- Caffeine. Although it's never mentioned in advertisements, caffeine is often that "extra ingredient" found in many combination pain relievers because it enables the drug to work more quickly.

These drugs can be an effective treatment, especially for mild to moderate migraines. A study of 1,357 migraine patients published in March, 1998, in the *Archives of Neurology,* found that of those who took a popular nonprescription headache remedy comprised of acetaminophen, aspirin and caffeine, 59 percent found their symptoms were eased, as compared to 33 percent who were given a placebo. After six hours, the number had risen to 79 percent compared to the 52 percent who took the placebo. The treatment relieved nausea and light-sensitivity as well.

But over-the-counter remedies do have drawbacks. Once upon a time, these "over-the-counter" medications were exactly that; they were handed to you over the counter by a pharmacist who knew and could advise you. Nowadays, though, we are likely to pick up these drugs at the supermarket. In this way, "over the counter" has become "off the shelf." Too often, we pop these pills without a thought.

There are a couple of problems with this approach. First, we too often assume that, if a drug is available without a prescription, it's free of side effects. That's not necessarily the case. Nonprescription drugs can be potent, especially these days, as more and more drugs which originally required a prescription are now available without one.

In fact, many of these drugs do have side effects. "The belief that over-the-counter medications are harmless is exactly what gets headache patients in trouble," warns Robert W. Rosum, a registered pharmacist who works with the New England Center for Headache in Stamford, Connecticut.

What is one of the best ways you can protect yourself? Follow this simple advice: Read the Label! Too often, we just down these pills without even checking the label. Remember that old edict, "Take two aspirin and call me in the morning"? That may be true of aspirin, but not necessarily for all the new extra-strength and combination pills lining the store shelves. Many of these drugs have very specific instructions that you can only find out about by reading the label.

Since nonprescription drugs are often the first line of defense against migraine, Dr. Fred D. Sheftell, who has written extensively on migraine, offers these recommendations:

> When it comes to warding off moderate tension-type headaches (and some migraineurs do also get tension headaches), a dose of one of the "simple" analgesics, such as aspirin, acetaminophen, or an NSAID, may prove sufficient. If it's not, the dosage can be repeated. You should follow the label's dosing or, if you wish to increase it, check with your doctor. Don't exceed the label's guidelines without your doctor's approval. Read the labels carefully, and pay attention to warnings that involve side effects or drug interactions. NSAIDs and ibuprofen can cause gastrointestinal bleeding which, in very rare cases, can be severe. They shouldn't be taken by people who have severe ulcer disease or certain types of gastrointestinal or bowel disease. NSAIDS should also be used cautiously by people with asthma. Drinking alcohol while you're taking acetaminophen can cause liver damage.

Remember, exercise caution, even though these drugs are obtainable with a prescription. It's possible for drug interactions to occur. Also, nonprescription drugs can cause headache rebound. It's also easy to lose track of how much nonprescription medicine you're taking. Keep track. Use your Migraine Calendar to stay aware of what you're taking—and how much of it.

#22

Choose the Right Drugs to Stop Migraine

There is nothing more important to a migraine sufferer than stopping an attack immediately. Abortive drugs are used to halt attacks, so here's a rundown on those that are available, both with and without prescriptions.

When it comes to stopping an attack, timing is all-important. Very early in the attack, mild medications, including nonprescription drugs, may do the trick. But even the most powerful drug may be useless if you wait too long. So if you sense a migraine coming on, stop what you're doing and take measures to treat it.

Analgesics

Nonprescription analgesics, including aspirin, acetaminophen, and NSAIDs, were dealt with in the previous chapter. There are, however, many prescription pain relievers used for migraine. They include prescription-strength naproxen (Naprosyn), naproxen sodium (Anaprox, Anaprox DS), mefenamic acid (Ponstel), and indomethacin (Indocin), to name a few.

ERGOTAMINES

Derived from a fungus, the ergotamine drugs have a powerful constricting effect on the blood vessels, preventing them from swelling. The common names for these drugs include Cafergot, Wigraine, and Ergostat. The most common, ergotamine tartrate, is available in tablets and suppository form. Suppositories are useful for those whose migraines include nausea and vomiting. Since these drugs themselves can bring on nausea and vomiting, antinausea drugs are often given with them.

Among those who should not take these drugs are those who are pregnant or planning to become pregnant, those with uncontrolled high blood pressure, cardiovascular disease, or liver or kidney disease. People using sumatriptan also shouldn't use them.

Ergotamine drugs can abort migraines, when used judiciously, and can also treat menstrual migraine. But they shouldn't be used daily because of the possibility of severe *rebound headaches*. Overusage of ergotamine can also be toxic, resulting in serious side effects, including heart attack, heart valve disease, and gangrene. People who become dependent on it may also suffer withdrawal; symptoms include severe headache, sweating, anxiety, and a rapid heartbeat. After withdrawal, though, the ergotamine-induced headaches eventually stop for most people, although the underlying migraine may remain.

ISOMETHEPTENE MUCATE COMBINATIONS

These drugs, when used in combination with acetaminophen and dichloralphenazone, act differently in the body from the ergotamine drugs but also cause the brain's blood vessels to constrict. They are used most often in children or those who cannot tolerate ergotamine. Their major side effect is dizziness, although drowsiness and gastrointestinal symptoms can also occur. These drugs shouldn't be taken more than three times a week. The drugs include Midrin and Isocom.

BARBITURATE COMPOUNDS

Barbiturates are central nervous system depressants, so they have a sedative effect. The combination drugs, which contain a short-acting barbiturate, along with aspirin or acetaminopehen, are often used by migraineurs who find that over-the-counter remedies do not help. They are most helpful when used in the early stages of migraine, but since they can cause a brief high or euphoria, they shouldn't be used to relieve stress or anxiety, because they can be habit-forming. If you've been taking these drugs regularly for a long time, do not stop without talking with your doctor. Side effects can include drowsiness, and they can enhance the effect of alcohol and other depressant drugs. These drugs include Fiorinal, Fioricet, Phrenilin, and Axotal.

NARCOTICS

When used sparingly, these drugs, also known as opiates, can be very effective in treating migraines that don't respond to weaker medications. These powerful pain relievers mimic the pain-suppressing chemicals found naturally in the body, called endorphins. Percocet, Percodan, codeine, Darvon, Vicodin, Lortabs, Stadol NS (a nasal spray), and Hydrocet are all narcotics. Side effects include sedation, dizziness, a drugged feeling, and confusion. Because these drugs have a history of being abused, doctors may be reluctant to prescribe them. But they shouldn't be ruled out for the treatment of migraine, writes Dr. Dewey Ziegler, of the University of Kansas Medical Center, in an article published in 1997 in *Neurologic Clinics*. He writes that these drugs should be given to migraine sufferers who cannot find relief any other way, and that their danger of overuse is more likely in people who get frequent tension headaches than in those who use them to stop specific migraine attacks.

DIHYDROERGOTAMINE (D.H.E. 45)

This drug, which belongs to the same class as ergotamine, is thought to work by affecting the serotonin system in the brain, constricting blood vessels and reducing inflammation. Since it can relieve migraine pain when an attack is at its height, it is a staple in the emergency treatment of migraine. It is available in a nasal spray by injection, in suppository form, or intravenously in hospitals. Drugs to counteract nausea or anxiety, which are side effects of dihydroergotamine, are often given as well.

CORTICOSTEROIDS

Cortisone, a strong anti-inflammatory drug given either by pill or injection, is one of the most effective treatments for severe, prolonged migraine, but it can only be used on a short-term basis because continual use can lead to bone loss, diabetes, cataracts, high blood pressure, and other serious diseases. Pill forms include Decadron and Prednisone; Depo-Medrol and ACTH (adrenocorticotroic hormone) are given by injection.

SUMATRIPTAN (IMITREX)

Sumatriptan is the first drug developed specifically to treat migraines. It acts directly on the neurotransmitters in the brain, particularly serotonin, the one most implicated in causing migraine. Since sumatriptan and related drugs (known as the triptans) are so important in the treatment of migraine, the next chapter is devoted to them.

#23

INVESTIGATE THE MIGRAINE "WONDER DRUGS"

Marketed under the brand name Imitrex, sumatriptan has revolutionized migraine treatment. Available in self-injecting, pill, and nasal spray form, this drug has brought relief to many migraine sufferers who previously had little or no success with other treatments.

Consider Michael's story. Michael is afflicted with intractable migraines. An award-winning photographer, he worked as best he could within the limitations of his disease, knowing that at any time he could suddenly become violently ill with a blinding headache, nausea, and vomiting. Even if the powerful medications he took worked, the next day he'd be groggy and unable to work. As soon as he recovered, another headache would strike, and the vicious cycle would begin again.

With the advent of sumatriptan, those days are gone. Although Michael still gets migraines, he can work. "In the old days, a migraine would drag on for three days, followed by a few more days feeling groggy. Now, a migraine costs me maybe eight hours, and the rest of my time is productive."

Michael suffers from the most severe form of migraine; those with milder migraines who take sumatriptan find it can halt attacks almost as soon as they start. For many, indeed, sumatriptan has been virtually a wonder drug.

It works by mimicking the action of the neurotransmitter serotonin. Serotonin affects nerve cells by stimulating and interacting with various types of receptors, which in turn trigger certain responses in the cells. Unlike other migraine medications, sumatriptan selectively activates the receptors that constrict blood vessels in the head, which are thought to be abnormally widened during a migraine attack.

Although it has been in use for relatively few years, many studies attest to the efficacy of sumatriptan. Generally, these studies show that, on average, 70 percent of migraine sufferers are able to return to their normal activities not long after taking the medication. Here are a few examples of some of the studies.

An article in *Neurology* published in 1996 looked at 453 migraine patients who used the drug over a two-year period. The study found that sumatriptan provided relief in at least two-thirds of the attacks of 85 percent of the patients. Another study, published that year in *Headache*, looked at sumatriptan in forty-three men and women. The study found that sumatriptan relieved migraine in 75 percent of these patients, compared with 25 percent who experienced relief using their usual therapy. Those taking sumatriptan also missed work less often and were able to return to their usual activities sooner. They also rated their quality of life higher than did those not using the drug. Other studies have found similar results.

But experiences with sumatriptan vary widely. Another study published in September 1996 in *Headache* found that nearly 20 percent of those who took the drug orally reported no relief. One problem is that the drug has a short life within the body, so the migraines can reoccur, as Barbara discovered.

"Imitrex gave me relief initially," says Barbara. After taking the drug, she experienced a few hours in which her headache seemed to vanish. However, she says, "it always came back with a vengeance after four to six hours."

Alison took the drug. She says, "It seems I was hit with every possible side effect, so I decided this wouldn't work for me."

And Marie found that, for her, Imitrex didn't work at all.

Sumatriptan should be used only for people who have been definitely diagnosed as suffering from migraine. It will not work for other types of headaches.

It's a very potent drug, so it's not the right choice for people who get very frequent migraines. And there are short-acting side effects. The most common side effects are pain at the injection site, tingling, a warm feeling all over, heaviness, and a sensation of pressure.

As noted, one key problem is that often the headache reoccurs. A study published in 1996 in *Cephalalgia* looked at 869 migraine patients who had used the drug for over two years and found that this occurred often, even when some people took a second dose. In fact, recurrent headache was also the major reason for stopping sumatriptan use.

Because it causes constriction of the blood vessels, sumatriptan shouldn't be used by people with heart disease or those who are at risk for it. Because it can cause constriction of the cardiovascular system, it's often recommended that patients take their first dose of sumatriptan in a physician's office or emergency room. In addition, if chest heaviness occurs, it is recommended the patient undergo cardiac tests to make sure there is no problem. People with a history of asthma or multiple drug allergies are also at increased risk of a potentially serious drug reaction. Furthermore, sumatriptan also should not be used within twenty-four hours of taking a drug containing ergot, such as Cafergot, or ergotamine derivatives such as D.H.E. 45. It is also not recommended for pregnant women.

The time at which sumatriptan is taken also appears to be

important. If it's taken too early, during the aura phase of a migraine, it will not prevent or relieve the subsequent headache. This is because the mechanism by which sumatriptan acts seems to be effective only when the headache has fully developed. This is in line with the view that sumatriptan acts at the very end of the cascade of events that results in migraine pain, not on the initial migraine trigger.

In the study published in *Headache* mentioned earlier, researchers tried to tease out why sumatriptan doesn't work in most people, but they could find no significant differences. They found, though, that those who didn't respond to the injection form tended to weigh more, had begun having migraines at an earlier age, and took the drug earlier in the course of their migraine. Those who didn't respond to the tablets had more vomiting and light sensitivity with their migraines, went to sleep more often after taking the drug, and more often experienced an initial worsening of headache after taking it.

It's important to learn which dosage is right for you. Leah first began taking Imitrex by injection, but after a while the nature of her migraines seemed to change, and the drug lost its effectiveness. She had also grown to dislike the injection process. When Imitrex became available in pill form, she decided to give it another try. However, she said, "I gave up on the pills too because they didn't seem effective as prescribed by my doctor." Eventually, though, Leah changed doctors. Her new doctor increased the dose and, she says, "I find now I do get relief from my headaches, even though it's for only ten to twelve hours at a time. My headaches last for three to five days, so I have to repeat taking it, but it's wonderful to have Imitrex back in my arsenal," she says.

Another drawback is that Imitrex is expensive. This can be a factor for people who pay for their prescriptions themselves or for those in managed health plans that seek to restrict the use of expensive drugs. "If you're on one of those insurance programs where you co-pay a few dollars for a prescription no matter what it's for, you get very indifferent to the price. However, each of the injections was $35, and for me it's never less than two. That makes a headache quite an expensive ordeal," noted Tom, a freelance writer.

It isn't only patients who are concerned about the price of Imitrex; insurers and managed health care plans sometimes balk at the cost as well. For more about this issue, see Chapter 49.

Although sumatriptan was the first of its kind, drug companies have developed different versions of this classification of drugs, including ones they hope will have fewer side effects. In fact, said Richard Lipton, codirector of the Montefiore Medical Center in the Bronx, New York, "we are moving into a world where choice will explode with the approval of the new triptans."

Imitrex was the first of these drugs; other triptans now available, under development or awaiting FDA approval, are Eletriptan, Naratriptan, Rizatriptan, and Zolomitriptan. Hopefully, these versions of sumatriptan will have fewer side effects and will be able to be given more widely. This is an area of migraine treatment you should watch carefully.

#24

CONSIDER PREVENTATIVE DRUGS

Tara doesn't have any heart problems, so when her doctor suggested that she take a cardiac drug to prevent her migraines, the idea struck her as odd. But now she finds herself impressed.

"I'm taking it daily and it's working! I've had only three minor migraines in the past month, compared to at least one migraine a week, which usually progressed to a major knockout," says the twenty-six-year-old marketing executive.

As a migraineur, your first priority should be to find a drug that offers you effective relief from attacks. But since your goal is also to reduce the number of attacks you get, preventative drugs can also play an important role. Usually these are drugs that you take daily. They are taken *in addition to the abortive drugs* for the relief of migraine attacks.

You may be a good candidate for preventative drugs if:

- You get migraines frequently, at least two or three times a month or more.
- Your migraines are incapacitating.

- You're psychologically unable to cope with your migraines.
- If abortive drugs don't work, or you can't take them due to side effects or other medical problems.

Writing in the journal *Neurologic Clinic* in 1997, Peer Tfelt-Hansen, M.D., noted that these are not hard and fast rules. For example, he notes, even a person who gets only one migraine a month may be a candidate for preventative drugs if that attack is very severe and disabling. Not all experts, though, agree with this view.

There are several types of preventative drugs. These drugs were developed to treat other diseases but coincidentally have been found to reduce migraines.

There are several important things to bear in mind.

First, preventative drugs don't affect migraines quickly. In fact, since it can take up to a few months to determine whether they work, many people discontinue taking them too soon. On the other hand, a doctor may encourage a patient to continue taking them even though they're ineffective. And, once you find something that works, your body may build up a tolerance to it, and you may have to change.

Second, preventative medications are intended to reduce the frequency or severity of migraines, but they don't completely eradicate them. That's why an abortive medication to handle the breakthrough migraine attacks is needed.

Third, the overuse of pain relievers, even over-the-counter ones, can render preventative drugs useless.

Fourth, these drugs shouldn't be used by women who are pregnant or planning to become so, because of their potential to harm the fetus.

Remember, even if you tried a preventative drug before and it didn't help, don't necessarily rule it out. Even trying the same drug again might work this time, especially if you were overusing pain relievers before.

How Are Preventative Drugs Prescribed?

In trying preventative medications, doctors usually start with a low dose and gradually increase it over a period of weeks until it begins to work. Generally, migraineurs tend to respond to low doses of medication, and they are also more likely to be sensitive to side effects, which can make it more difficult for them to keep taking a drug, even if it is effective.

These drugs don't necessarily need to be used forever. Sometimes preventative medications can be stopped or reduced after the migraines are well controlled, and the improvement will continue.

Which Drug Should You Use?

Choosing among the many preventative drugs is not an easy task; indeed, it is a complex one in which the benefits of the drug are weighed against the potential side effects.

When prescribing preventative drugs, your doctor will consider not only your migraines but other diseases you may have. This is because a single drug can be used to improve more than one condition, but side effects must be taken into consideration. For example, a beta blocker can treat both migraine and high blood pressure, but it can also cause depression, so it's not a good choice for someone prone to this ailment. Therefore, giving your doctor a complete accounting of your medical history is imperative.

Preventative drugs are generally prescribed one at a time, but they can be combined for specific results. One example of this is the pairing of the antidepressant amitriptyline (Elavil) with the beta blocker propranolol (Inderal). Inderal lowers the pulse rate, but Elavil raises the heart rate to counteract this effect.

In prescribing preventative drugs, the following medical conditions should be taken into account:

- Cardiovascular disorders, including heart disease or a history of stroke
- Mood disorders, including depression, manic depression, anxiety, or panic attacks
- Gastrointestinal problems
- Allergies
- Asthma
- Epilepsy

Here's a rundown on the most popular drugs used to prevent migraine.

BETA BLOCKERS

Years ago, a patient in South Africa who was taking a beta blocker, propranolol (Inderal), for his heart condition, reported that his longstanding migraines had disappeared. His doctor wrote up the findings, which led to the first controlled study of the drug in 1972. Since then, a number of other drugs in this class have been found to be migraine preventatives, including nadolol (Corgard), metoprolol (Lopressor), atenolol (Tenormin), and timolol (Blocadren).

Beta blockers act by blocking the action of certain substances, including adrenaline, to lower heart rate and blood pressure. They may act on migraines by preventing the dilation, or widening, of blood vessels. Side effects, which occur in about 10 to 15 percent of people, include fatigue, cold hands and feet, and dizziness. There are also side effects that affect the central nervous system, including vivid dreams, nightmares, night hallucinations, insomnia, and depression. To minimize the possibility of side effects, beta blockers are usually begun at low doses and increased gradually.

The amount of beta blocker needed to be effective can vary greatly, so dosages should be individually calculated. It's generally agreed that anyone taking beta blockers—migraineurs included—shouldn't stop taking them abruptly but should instead reduce the amount they're taking gradually.

Migraineurs who experience auras may not be good candidates for beta blockers. And they are not advised for people with certain diseases—asthma or chronic obstructive lung disease, congestive heart failure, certain other types of heart problems, diabetes, low blood sugar, a too slow heart, low blood pressure, Raynaud's disease, peripheral vascular disease, or severe depression.

Calcium Channel Blockers

These drugs act by stabilizing the cranial blood vessels and preventing their expansion, believed to be a factor in causing migraines. Some studies have found them more useful in treating cluster headaches, but some migraineurs find them quite effective. Verapamil (Calan, Isoptin, and Verelan) has been found to be the most effective for migraine.

The most common side effects are constipation and fluid retention. Although they are used to treat heart problems, people with congestive heart failure or certain types of heartbeat irregularities shouldn't use them. They are also not used in combination with beta blockers. Men attempting to father children shouldn't use them because they reduce penetration of the egg by the sperm.

Nonsteroidal Anti-Inflammatory Drugs (NSAIDS)

If you've found NSAIDs, such as those discussed in the "over-the-counter" section, to be an effective abortive medication for relieving your migraines, your doctor may prescribe them as a daily, preventative medication.

Aspirin, in daily doses ranging from 300 to 600 milligrams, and naproxen sodium, both in its prescription form and its non-prescription form, Aleve, are examples of NSAIDs used for migraine prevention. Other NSAIDs are effective as well. They can be used on a long-term basis as long as they don't cause ulcers or blood thinning, which can be indicated by easy bruising. People with ulcers, those on blood-thinning drugs, or people with liver or kidney disease shouldn't take them. They also shouldn't be used in children younger than twelve years of age.

ANTIDEPRESSANTS

Just as migraineurs can be surprised when they're prescribed a cardiac drug, they also may be taken aback if their doctor prescribes an antidepressant. But such drugs can prevent migraines, although they're usually given in doses smaller than those used to treat depression.

It's believed that antidepressants reduce the frequency of migraines by manipulating the levels of certain chemicals in the blood, particularly the neurotransmitter serotonin. The three categories of antidepressants used for migraine prevention are the tricyclic antidepressants, the selective serotonin reuptake inhibitors (SSRIs), and the monoamine oxidase inhibitors (MAOIs).

The most prominent among the tricyclic antidepressants used for migraine prevention is amitriptyline (Elavil). Others that are often used include doxepin (Sinquan, Adapin) and nortriptyline (Pamelor, Aventyl). These drugs are usually taken at bedtime because they are designed to help people with sleep disorders. Their side effects may include weight gain, dry mouth, blurred vision, urine retention, and sexual dysfunction. These drugs also should not be taken by people who have heartbeat irregularities, narrow-angle glaucoma, or urinary problems, or by pregnant or breast-feeding women.

SSRIs, a newer type of treatment, include fluoxetine (Prozac), sertraline (Zoloft), and paroxetine (Paxil). These drugs have fewer side effects than the older antidepressants, but their effectiveness in reducing migraines is still being researched.

MAOIs comprise a potent class of antidepressants that can help those who suffer from very severe migraines where other preventative medications have failed. But since those who take them must follow strict dietary rules and restrict their use of certain medicines, they are prescribed very cautiously. They also carry their own side effects, including insomnia, weight gain, and changes in blood pressure. Phenelzine (Nardil) and isocarboxazid (Marplan) are examples of MAOIs.

ANTISEROTONIN AGENTS

The oldest of these drugs, methysergide (Sansert), is thought to work by blocking serotonin receptors, preventing inflammation in the brain and the narrowing of the blood vessels. However, because of its potential for serious side effects, it's generally only used when other preventative drugs haven't worked.

Many people experience increased appetite and sleepiness; other side effects include nausea, vomiting, stomach discomfort, swelling, dizziness, and depression.

Long-term users may develop a serious problem involving the overgrowth of connective tissue among various organs; therefore, people taking this drug are often told to take a drug holiday of a month or so to make sure this isn't occurring. They are tapered off the drug, though, so rebound headache doesn't occur.

People who shouldn't take this type of drug include those with heart disease, severe high blood pressure, a history of blood clots, peptic ulcers, familial fibrotic disorders, lung diseases, or diseases of the connective tissue, liver, or kidneys.

If preventative drugs don't work for you, make sure you're taking them correctly. A 1994 study in *Cephalalgia* looked at nine migraineurs whose use of preventative drugs was measured by a device concealed in the container's lid. Five participants chose not to complete the study, and the remaining four took less than the dosages specified. So if you've decided to try preventative drugs, give them a fair chance. On the other hand, if you've given them a fair trial and they don't work, talk to your doctor about changing them. Sometimes even though one type of preventative drug doesn't work, another will.

#25

ELIMINATE REBOUND HEADACHES

One of the least-known, but most common, types of headache is rebound headache. The cause of this problem is the very substance taken to relieve it—headache medicine.

Surprised? You may well be. Although rebound headache is a common side effect of many medications, you won't learn about it from drug ads. But this problem is well known to headache experts, who frequently see sufferers using too much medication and unwittingly setting themselves up for this type of headache.

Drug rebound doesn't cause migraine attacks. However, it can cause migraineurs to develop additional headaches that can become indistinguishable from their migraines until they are experiencing head pain sometimes every day.

No one knows exactly how drugs cause rebound headache. One theory is that chronic overuse of these substances may interfere with the brain's ability to modulate pain. Another is that your body becomes so accustomed to a certain amount of pain reliever that if it falls too low, the result is a withdrawal headache.

How widespread is this problem? In a 1997 article in *Neurologic Clinics,* Dr. Fred Sheftell calls it "overwhelming." But because both sufferers and their doctors are often unaware of it, it escapes diagnosis.

It is not uncommon for tension headache sufferers to develop drug rebound. Because of the frequent nature of tension headaches, people with these headaches are inclined to overuse medication.

But migraine is a different problem. In most people, migraine attacks occur sporadically. A rebound problem signifies that the migraineur is not getting effective pain relief, so stronger drugs, or other measures, may be in order.

The unfortunate result of rebound is that a migraine problem that was once treatable becomes resistant. The natural course of the migraine is changed into a more intractable type known as chronic daily headache (CDH). When this occurs in migraineurs, it's known as transformed migraine.

There are other ramifications as well. Chronic overuse of pain relievers also lowers the pain threshold in sufferers, resulting in more frequent headaches and worse pain. In addition, although it is not understood why, overusing these drugs can make the use of preventative medications ineffective.

In another article published in 1997 in *Neurologic Clinics,* Ninan T. Mathew, M.D., described the clinical features of rebound headaches. They include:

- Headaches that occur daily or nearly daily
- Headaches that occur in headache sufferers who take pain relievers very frequently, often in excessive amounts
- Headaches that vary in the severity, type, and location of pain

- Headaches that appear in people who seem to have a low threshold for pain.
- Headaches accompanied by fatigue, nausea, stomach distress, restlessness, anxiety, irritability, memory problems, difficulty concentrating, and depression
- Headaches that occur in the early morning hours, between 2 and 5 A.M.
- Headaches that worsen over time, necessitating larger and more frequent doses of drugs
- Headache symptoms that appear when medication is discontinued abruptly

If you assume that you would notice if headache rebound was happening to you, think again. This situation can occur so subtly and in a way so seemingly unrelated to the medication, you may not even notice it.

Experts disagree over whether aspirin and NSAIDs can cause headache rebound, but they concur that many other types of pain relievers can. This especially includes those containing caffeine, such as Anacin and Excedrin, and drugs combined with codeine. Prescription drugs that can cause this problem include barbiturate-based combination drugs—such as Fiorinal, Fioricet, and Esgic—and narcotic-based combination drugs, such as Percocet, Tylox, and Vicodin. Ergotamine tartrate can lead not only to serious rebound headache but also to a potentially dangerous condition known as lead ergotism, a disorder that can lead to organ damage and even death. There is disagreement over the subject of narcotics; sometimes articles describing rebound blur the issue by talking about both analgesics and narcotics. (As noted earlier, narcotics can be taken safely by migraineurs to relieve sporadic, severe attacks.)

If you're experiencing rebound headache, you need to be withdrawn from the medication. Such a withdrawal period can take months. Withdrawing from these drugs won't relieve all your headaches—just the ones caused by rebound. But it will make implementing an effective migraine management program feasible.

If the problem is over-the-counter drugs, you may be able to taper off by yourself. Be prepared for some very bad headaches. Since most sufferers fear this the most, such withdrawal may be too difficult to attempt alone. Your doctor can help by prescribing certain medications that can get you through this period without exacerbating your rebound problem.

If you're using prescription drugs, or you have other problems, such as anxiety or depression, you should be withdrawn under medical supervision. If you've become dependent on pain relievers that contain barbiturates, you may have to be withdrawn more gradually to avoid such symptoms as seizures. If you're suffering from CDH that's resistant to treatment, you may need to be given D.H.E. 45 intravenously.

Once you're no longer taking the pain relievers, you and your doctor can work together to implement an effective migraine management plan. Such a plan may include abortive medication for attacks, possibly a preventative drug, and possibly a program of behavioral methods such as biofeedback. Education about the proper use of medication is also a must.

Remember, rebound headache is a common but serious and insidious problem that can scuttle the best attempts to treat migraine. It is sometimes even overlooked by doctors. If you suspect you may have this problem, getting treatment will be the best thing you can do to find effective migraine relief.

#26

PREPARE FOR EMERGENCY ROOM TRIPS

It was a hot July day, and Kristen felt a migraine coming on. But this time, as the hours passed, her head pain worsened. She began to feel tingling on the left side of her body and, eventually, it became numb. Frightened, she called her doctor. After reviewing her symptoms, her doctor recommended she go to her local hospital emergency room. After performing several neurological tests, the doctor determined that Kristen was, indeed, suffering from migraine, not anything else.

It would be ideal if all migraines could be treated at home. But the truth is that sometimes migraine patients need to go to the emergency room as a last resort. And there are legitimate reasons to go. They are:

- If you're experiencing head pain that's worse than any you've ever had before
- If you're experiencing head pain that is changing in nature and severe

- If you're experiencing head pain that worsens progressively over days or weeks
- If your head pain is associated with fever, stiff neck, or other illness
- If you've suffered a head injury or some other trauma

Sometimes, too, sufferers end up at the emergency room when they're suffering from a severe, incapacitating migraine, their medication offers no relief, and they've reached the end of their ability to cope.

These are all sound reasons to head for an emergency room.

Sometimes, you'll receive compassionate help. But it's also an unfortunate fact that sometimes emergency room personnel can be unreceptive to migraine sufferers. Often, problems arise if a migraineur arrives at the emergency room and requests (or demands) certain drugs. This can be a warning flag to hospital personnel who have been trained to be on the lookout for drug addicts. And many emergency room doctors are not well trained in the treatment of migraine and may treat sufferers indifferently.

Ideally, an emergency room will have personnel who are sensitive to the fact that migraineurs' attacks are made worse by noise and light. Hopefully, you'll be taken into a quiet room where a medical history will be taken and you'll be given a brief physical and neurological examination. If there are warning signs that you may be suffering from a problem other than migraine, a more extensive examination, including blood tests and possibly an emergency CT scan, may also be warranted. Once the diagnosis of migraine is made, you'll be treated and sent home. What type of treatment you'll receive will depend on the type of problem.

There are certain medications that are only available in an emergency room. Among the most popular is dihydroergotamine, known also as D.H.E. 45, administered intravenously or by injection (a nasal spray is available for home use). It is given alone or with accompanying medications to prevent nausea and anxiety. Sumatriptan, although obtainable for use at home, is another popular abortive migraine medication offered in emergency settings. For patients who cannot take sumatriptan or D.H.E. 45, there are other medications that can be given intravenously, including prochlorperazine (Compazine), chlorpromazine (Thorazine), and sometimes tranquilizers. Narcotics are offered very cautiously because of their addictive potential. These would include meperidine (Demerol), morphine, and butorphanol (Stadol). There are several antinausea medications that can be used as well.

If you visit the emergency room, Dr. Merle Diamond, of the Diamond Headache Clinic, offers these steps you can take to enhance the likelihood that you will receive the help—and compassion—you need.

First, prepare for the eventuality that sometimes you'll need emergency help. If you're seeing a doctor for the first time, approach this subject as part of the discussion of your migraines. You can explain to the doctor that, occasionally, you've found it necessary to go to the emergency room. Ask your doctor to call the hospital when you need emergency treatment. Such a call usually allays the emergency room doctor's concerns and lends your complaint credibility. If you are traveling, request a letter from your doctor that you can show the emergency room physician.

When you arrive at the emergency room, be calm. Relate the history of your headaches, the tests you have had, the medications you commonly take, and the steps you took to combat your migraine this time. Emergency room staff can be suspicious when a patient presents a lengthy drug history, but if you discuss it in relation to your migraine history, this can help allay their concern. Prepare this information ahead of time, so you don't have to try and recall it when you're in the midst of a migraine.

Bring someone with you, as you may be given strong medications that will make you so groggy that you'll need someone to drive you home.

In these days of more and more restricted health care, you may find it difficult to get your health insurance company to pay for your emergency room treatment. This issue is covered in a later chapter.

PART FIVE

MANAGING MIGRAINE WITHOUT DRUGS

#27

INVESTIGATE ALTERNATIVE TREATMENTS

Much of this book contains the most up-to-date information that can be gleaned from conventional medicine. This is traditional, Western medicine, founded by Hippocrates, which has come to rely on the scientific method of clinical testing as the cornerstone for evaluating effectiveness.

But migraine is a complex disease that may need to be fought on more than one battleground. Many people are unable to take drugs because of their side effects, or they prefer not to. Fortunately, there are some methods that do not call for drugs that have been known to be effective. Only the treatments that have been shown to be the most effective in treating migraines are included in this book. They include biofeedback, stress reduction, and, to lesser degrees, relaxation and meditation.

Eastern medicine has also played a part in migraine treatment. The goal of traditional Eastern medicine is to stimulate the body's own healing abilities. A variety of methods fall under the heading of Eastern medicine. Acupuncture and the herb feverfew are examples.

Which is more effective, drug or nondrug therapy? This is an important question, but not many studies have been done comparing the two, so no firm conclusions can be drawn. However, a study published in 1994 in *Behavioral Medicine* compared the results of trials using propranolol (Inderal), the most popular migraine preventative, with the use of biofeedback. The study found that both treatments reduced the occurrence of migraine by about 50 percent. The article goes on to note, however, that preventative drugs might be necessary to manage more severe and complicated headache problems.

Because migraine is a complex disease, its treatment need not be a "one-or-the-other" approach. For migraine particularly, it's been found that neither traditional nor nontraditional medicine alone works for everyone. Migraine is a challenging disease that may require not a single bullet but an arsenal of weapons. Whether you opt for conventional or alternative medicine may be a matter of your philosophy. But many migraineurs find their greatest success in using a combination of methods.

#28

Learn the Truth About Stress

Excruciating migraines are bad enough, but getting blamed for bringing the ailment on yourself can be even worse, says Michael John Coleman, executive director of Migraine Awareness Group: A National Understanding For Migraine (M.A.G.N.U.M.). He notes that, although it's now agreed that migraine is a biological illness, many magazines, newspaper articles and even books still characterize stress as the chief cause of migraine. This brings even more heartache to the migraine sufferers, who are wrongly blamed—or blame themselves—for their attacks.

"We now know that migraine is a disease. We know that stress doesn't cause migraine. But stress is a big factor in the migraineur's life and a lot of this stress comes from being told, by their family and friends, that they cannot handle life. Stress isn't good, but blaming migraine on stress is like blaming the victim," says Coleman.

Stress used to be considered the major cause of migraine. Nowadays, this is known to be a myth amongst most in the scientific community. Instead, stress is portrayed not as the major cause of migraines, but as a possible contributing factor. It's very hard for most people to draw a distinction between a "cause" and a "contributor," so the myth about stress sticks.

But the idea that migraineurs can't handle stress has some large holes in it.

First, consider the fact that most migraineurs don't have attacks when they're under stress, but usually after the stressful period has abated. Leah, for example, is typical of many. "I've had many occasions in which I've had to prepare for countless meetings and conference presentations and talks for corporate executives. At home, I've had up to three hundred dinner guests. I find that, when I'm preparing for these events and executing them, I'm headache free. It's not until afterwards that the crashing blows of a full migraine descend upon me," she says.

Second, the vast majority of migraineurs continue to function in their lives, despite being beset by the most excruciatingly painful and debilitating attacks, as well as the threat that hangs over them that they could suffer another one anytime. This would seem to demonstrate that migraineurs are at least as emotionally strong as anyone else, possibly even more so.

Third, consider the growing genetic evidence and the imaging tests which track brain changes which occur during migraine. It becomes increasingly evident that migraine is primarily a biological, not a psychological, problem.

Given all that, however, there are some ways in which stress may impact migraine. Consider these points:

First, although stress doesn't cause migraine, it does cause tension headaches, and many migraineurs experience both. In fact, a study published in the journal *Pain* found that migraineurs who also get tension headaches suffer longer ones. So, if you get tension headaches, learning to manage stress can relieve at least some of the head pain you suffer.

Second, stress causes physiological changes in the body's nervous system, including a rise in heart rate, blood pressure, and the release of certain hormones. It's believed that the autonomic nervous system of migraineurs may be physiologically hypersensitive to such changes, although the resulting migraines are usually experienced after the stressful event is over.

Third, contending with a disease which is as misunderstood as migraine is inherently stressful in itself. Learning to manage this stress may help you contend with all the people you encounter in life who simply do not understand the pain you endure.

#29

TRY THESE ANTISTRESS STRATEGIES

Here, in brief, are a few strategies to help you relieve stress on the job and at home. More formal stress management techniques are discussed in the next chapter.

STRETCH

If you sit at a desk for long periods of time, stand up and take a stretch. Frequent breaks will ease your neck and scalp muscles. Get up, stretch, walk around a bit. Shrug your shoulders and bend your neck. Some people find that specially designed computer keyboards can help.

TAKE A "VIRTUAL VACATION"

For most of us, it's impossible to take frequent long vacations. But using only your imagination, you can take frequent mini-vacations. This is done via a technique called visualization, a rather fancy name for what used to simply be called daydreaming. Close your eyes; imagine your favorite vacation spot. Is it the beach? You're lying there—isn't the sun warm? Or perhaps you're flying down your favorite ski slope; can't you feel the fresh, cool air on your face—or can't you see your hair fly as you sail along in your boat? Even a five- or ten-minute "virtual vacation" can leave you feeling surprisingly refreshed.

PAMPER YOURSELF

Sometimes in our stress-filled days it's easy to cram in too much and neglect being good to yourself. Whether you're a man or a woman, pampering yourself can reduce your stress, which hopefully will help prevent migraines as well. Treat yourself to a quiet hour with a good book, see a movie, or take a long walk.

MEDITATE

Meditation is a process in which one tries to achieve awareness without thought. Depending on your personality, there are two different types of meditation that might appeal to you. In Transcendental Meditation (TM), which was popularized by the Maharishi Mahesh Yogi in the United States in the 1970s, practitioners focus on and mentally repeat a short phrase called a mantra. Practitioners of mindfulness meditation learn to pay close moment-to-moment attention to whatever is going on in their minds. Mindfulness meditation is directed toward learning to live in the present and is an excellent way to not only reduce stress but also eliminate unnecessary worrying.

YOGA

Relaxation, deep breathing, meditation, and stretching your body are all stress reducers. Yoga, a system of Hindu philosophy and religion, combines all four.

The form of yoga most familiar to Westerners is hatha

yoga, in which the practitioner assumes a series of poses, known as asanas, and uses a special breathing technique. These exercises maintain flexibility and teach physical and mental control.

In addition, yoga practitioners learn the type of deep abdominal breathing that is the foundation of many relaxation methods. In using breathing, yoga followers also are encouraged to clear their minds and let their thoughts go, practices shared by all meditators.

If you're considering yoga, you should make sure the person who teaches you is qualified. For more information, see the Resources section.

Laugh Once a Day (At Least)

There's nothing funny about migraines. But focusing on illness and pain can sap your joy in life. One of the best ways to regain it is to laugh—at least once a day. Although laughter is thought of as a emotional response, it has physiological effects as well. It's been found that, after a good laugh, your blood pressure and heart rate decrease, leaving you very relaxed. Laughter also has been found to indirectly stimulate endorphins, the brain's natural painkillers.

#30

BREAK FREE OF MENTAL "STRAITJACKETS"

If your boss, who is standing in front of you, launches into a tirade, it's no mystery that this might cause stress, right? Well, no, and yes. On one hand, part of your stress is, of course, being generated by your boss. On the other, some of your stress may also come from what you're telling yourself as the tirade continues. "She's right, I should've done better." "I'm such a jerk." "No wonder she's angry."

These statements are examples of negative self-talk that exacerbates stress. If you're like most of us, you don't need that boss standing over you, telling you these things, to hear them; you do a good job telling them to yourself.

"Such negative self-talk is the root cause of unhealthy stress," notes Dr. Michael McKee. "Although it's a stressful world, the greatest cause of stress, in almost everyone, is ourselves. It is the kinds of beliefs we have and the kinds of rules we live by that really create stress."

Psychologists call one of the sources of negative self-talk straitjackets. These are the ironclad rules that shape our thoughts. We absorbed many of these principles as a child, before we could think for ourselves. These unconscious rules govern our behavior, even though they don't necessarily make sense.

For example, if you're a boy, you may have learned: "I have to be strong" or "Boys don't cry." Girls, on the other hand, learned talk like: "What are little girls made of? Sugar, spice, and everything nice."

Here are some other straitjackets:

- Anything worth doing is worth doing well.
- Finish what you start.
- It's terrible to make a mistake.
- Don't take the easy way out.
- Live up to your potential.

Getting rid of these straitjackets takes thought. The first step is recognizing them; the second is revising them. For example:

Anything worth doing is worth doing well.

Anything? Not necessarily. Certainly, it's important to do some things right; you wouldn't want to hire a slipshod contractor or electrician. But there are tasks in life which can be done in a quicker, less perfect manner, and still be perfectly satisfactory.

Finish what you start.

If you start a new hobby and don't like it, there's no shame in abandoning it and going on to something you prefer. Likewise, you don't need to finish that 400-page book that began boring you on page one.

It's terrible to make a mistake.

Everyone makes mistakes and many are harmless errors.

Don't take the easy way out.

Why not? Life can be difficult; why make it harder?

You must live up to your potential.

Potential? That's a very vague term, isn't it? How can you live up to something you can't even describe.

To rid yourself of these straitjackets, you need to examine your thoughts and learn the ones that you subconsciously subscribe to. Then, substitute a more freeing version, for example, *it's okay to finish something I've started if that is the best thing to do.* By consciously repeating the positive force, you will eventually supplant the negative ones, and free yourself of the straitjackets that encase you.

#31

TRY BIOFEEDBACK

Once considered only in the realm of alternative medicine, biofeedback has won increasing acceptance by the medical establishment as an effective treatment for a number of disorders, including migraine.

Biofeedback is a method by which you can learn to control bodily functions which are usually considered involuntary, including skin temperature, muscle contraction, heart rate, blood pressure and brain waves. Biofeedback training is done by a professional trainer using equipment to monitor your responses, but the goal is to teach you techniques that you can use at home. Learning biofeedback usually takes several sessions.

Traditionally, the type of biofeedback generally used for migraine is known as thermal biofeedback, which involves the regulation of skin temperature. When you're under stress, your blood vessels constrict, and your hands get cold. With this method, it's possible to raise the temperature in your hands, achieving a more relaxed state.

With biofeedback, usually sensors are attached to your body to provide visual and auditory signals that show the amount of tension which exists and how much relaxation is being achieved. This way, you receive immediate feedback on your success. You're usually also asked to keep a diary to measure the success of the practice.

Several studies have looked at the effect of biofeedback generally and found positive results. Among them was a study published in June 1995 in the journal *Headache*, which compared twenty-five migraineurs who were randomly assigned to biofeedback groups with those who relaxed on their own. The study found that those in the biofeedback group decreased their pain scores by 47 percent and their medication by 66 percent, while the groups practicing self-relaxation reported much smaller changes. This study confirmed a previous one involving twenty-three migraine patients published in the same journal the year before.

Biofeedback is considered different from more general relaxation techniques because its goal is to teach the practitioner to control specific bodily functions, not general relaxation. But it is often combined with other relaxation techniques, and this may offer the most effective relief. In a study published in 1994 in the journal *Behavioral Medicine*, researchers analyzed seventy-two studies which evaluated biofeedback and relaxation training. When those results were averaged, the combination of relaxation and biofeedback averaged better results than either therapy alone.

People who get migraines usually call upon their biofeedback training in different ways. Some use it at the first sign of an impending migraine attack, in hopes of warding it off. But it's also recommended as a daily preventative, to sooth the physical effects of stress.

It isn't known exactly how biofeedback helps migraine. There is a theory that migraineurs have "hypersensitive" nervous systems. This means that, although they are unaware of it, their nervous systems are more highly attuned to changes which occur throughout the day. It's thought that biofeedback helps such individuals "even out" these fluctuations.

If you're interested in exploring biofeedback, you can get a reference from the psychology department of a local university or a headache center, or check the Resources section.

#32

EXPERIENCE RELAXATION

Relaxation techniques are methods of consciously releasing muscular tension to achieve a state of mental calm. These techniques can help prevent migraines.

There are two categories of relaxation techniques. Active relaxation consists of alternately tensing and relaxing all of the muscles in your body. Passive relaxation involves clearing the mind to concentrate on a single phrase or sound. This is similar to meditation, which is described in Chapter 29.

Before you begin, remember these key points:

- You don't need to work hard at relaxing. Learning to relax is a skill, and you get better at a skill naturally, through practice.
- Trust your body. Don't monitor your thoughts too carefully; having your mind wander during relaxation is natural.
- Enjoy yourself. This may be the only time in the day

when you are concentrating on taking care of yourself. Enjoy this time; don't make it just more work!

Now, here's some summaries of popular relaxation techniques:

BECOMING AWARE OF YOUR BODY

Body awareness is training yourself to pay attention to your various bodily sensations. Michael G. McKee, Ph.D., of the Cleveland Clinic Foundation Department of Psychiatry and Psychology, suggests these simple exercises to train yourself to become more aware. For example, to train yourself to be more aware of your environment, he suggests completing the sentence "I am aware of _____." Example: "I am aware of the smell of coffee and the sound of a car passing by." To become aware of the physiological sensations in your body, complete the sentence "I feel _____." Example: "I feel hungry, my neck is stiff and my hands are clenched."

This technique enables you to identify how you react to various situations and learn how to put the relaxation techniques described in this section to good use.

ABDOMINAL BREATHING

Abdominal breathing is a very relaxed form of the activity we do all the time—breathing. However, breathing in this state is what we do when we're sleeping deeply. Here's an exercise to learn abdominal breathing:

1. Sit comfortably in a chair or lie on the floor. Put one hand over your chest and one hand over your stomach.
2. Breathing only through your nose, if possible, inhale slowly and evenly while gently moving your stomach

out. You should feel some tightening in your stomach when you reach full inhalation.

3. Let the breath go slowly through your nostrils. As you exhale, the hand on your stomach will go down and you will feel the tightness in your stomach disappear. Imagine, as you breathe out, that you are letting go of all the tension in your entire body.

SCANNING YOUR BODY

Body scanning is a process of scanning your body to find areas of tension. In doing so, you learn to differentiate and identify various levels of tension and how to relax these areas. To do this, lie on your back and move your mind through the different regions of the body, methodically working your way from your toes up to the top of your head, allowing your breathing to flow over your body at the same time. This is designed to relax all of your muscles and allow any tension to disappear. The idea is to literally feel each region, seeking out tension and, with your breathing, enabling it to flow out of your body. As you become proficient, you will no longer need to lie down to do this technique; you can practice it anywhere, at your desk, on an airplane, whenever you are feeling particularly pressured.

PROGRESSIVE MUSCLE RELAXATION (PMR)

This is an active form of relaxation that you do by alternately tensing, and relaxing, all of the major muscle groups in the body. PMR helps you learn what the major muscles and muscle groups are, focuses on how each muscle group feels when tense and relaxed, and shows you how to become more aware of how your body feels when you are tense. Since it is an active exercise, PMR is especially useful for people who find it difficult to sit still for an extended period of time. In short, if the idea of relaxing fills you with stress, PMR may fit the bill.

Check the Resources section to find books and tapes that can guide you through these and other stress management exercises.

#33

CONSIDER ACUPUNCTURE

Acupuncture is the insertion of thin needles into specific points of the body in order to prevent or treat illness. Long a staple of Eastern medicine, acupuncture is winning converts in the West for the treatment of many types of chronic pain, including migraine.

According to traditional Chinese medicine, acupuncture works by correcting the balance of energy, or qi, in the body. For good health, this flow of energy must move properly through the body, and disruptions in it can cause illness and pain. The insertion of acupuncture needles is done to correct such difficulties. By the way, if you are put off by the needles, acupressure is a similar technique using the operator's hands to press upon the body's pressure points.

In 1997 the National Institutes of Health convened a conference on acupuncture. After reviewing many studies, an independent panel concluded that acupuncture is an effective therapy for certain medical conditions and should be integrated into standard practice. The panel judged acupuncture effective in reducing nausea associated with pregnancy and cancer chemotherapy and pain following dental surgery. The report fell short of endorsing acupuncture for the treatment of all forms of pain but said that the evidence was promising in the area of headache; it called for more, larger studies. The separate issue of migraine was not addressed.

Why does acupuncture appear to work? Critics point to the placebo effect, the well-known phenomenon in which a treatment (or fake treatment) is effective simply because the patient believes in it. Another explanation is that the use of these needles stimulates the body to produce endorphins, the natural, narcoticlike substances produced by the brain.

There is some research to back up the use of acupuncture for migraines. A 1995 article in *Headache* reported on a study of twenty-six migraineurs (nineteen women and seven men). A majority, 66 percent, reported a 33 percent improvement after treatment, and this improvement continued for 58 percent of them for the three-year followup. Their need for medication was also reduced.

At the Cleveland Clinic Foundation, Dr. Ramesh Sogal, a staff anesthesiologist, pain therapist, and acupuncturist, uses acupuncture to treat all types of headache, migraine included.

When Dr. Sogal sees a patient, he performs an examination according to Chinese practice to try and determine if it is a problem in which acupuncture will be useful. He says the treatment lessens the frequency of migraines in some; others find that it helps the medications they are taking work more effectively.

Acupuncture patients at the Cleveland Clinic undergo ten sessions, each lasting about twenty minutes. Dr. Sogal notes that acupuncture is not "like a drug that works right away"; it takes about three or four treatments to produce an effect.

If you are considering acupuncture, it's very important that the practitioner use disposable needles. Check to see if the practitioner is certified. Not all states require licensing, but many do. If your state doesn't, choose an acupuncturist certified by the National Commission for the Certification of Acupuncturists. You can also find a doctor who is a certified acupuncturist by calling the American Academy of Medical Acupuncture.

#34

GROW FEVERFEW

When Rhoda senses she's getting a migraine, she goes out into the yard and grazes.

"I tend to get most of my migraines in the summer. I don't know why; perhaps it's the sun. But I go out in the yard, nibble a bit, and my headache is gone in about an hour," says Rhoda.

There is a long list of botanical herbs that are believed to imbue health, but when it comes to migraine, most of the attention has centered on feverfew, an herb very popular in England for the relief of migraine, which has been catching on in the United States as well.

Although it's not known exactly how feverfew works, it's believed that extracts from the plant inhibit the release of two substances that can cause inflammation in the brain's cells: the neurotransmitter serotonin and prostaglandin from the white blood cells.

In one study, reported in *The Lancet* in 1989, migraineurs were divided into two groups. One group received a daily capsule containing freeze-dried feverfew, the other a placebo. After two months, the groups were switched. The groups receiving the feverfew reported fewer migraines and less severe pain. Another study, published in the *British Medical Journal* a few years earlier, reported that 70 percent of 270 migraine sufferers who chewed feverfew leaves also reported improvement.

It's not clear, though, what is the best way to ingest feverfew. Many adherents, like Rhoda, favor eating the leaves. A bushy perennial, feverfew grows to about two feet and is laden with flowers. Of course, in the winter the leaves will die, so you can air-dry feverfew, crush it, and put it in a tightly capped bottle for later use.

Feverfew capsules are sold in health food stores, but there is no required standardization of herbal products, so the strength of prepared formulas can vary considerably.

In his book *The Headache Alternative: A Neurologist's Guide to Drug-Free Relief,* Dr. Alexander Mauskop notes that chewing two fresh or freeze-dried leaves gives you about 170 milligrams of feverfew; alternatively, he recommends 125 milligrams of prepared, dried feverfew that contains at least 0.2 percent parthenolide. He also cautions that you make sure the preparation or the fresh leaf is labeled "authenticated feverfew."

He also warns that although feverfew is relatively safe, it can cause mouth sores or stomach upset. The sores are not caused by the leaves: they've been experienced by those taking capsules as well. Some researchers say it shouldn't be taken by pregnant or breast-feeding women, and that you should consult your doctor if you wish to take it for more than four months in a row.

#35

CONSIDER THESE SUPPLEMENTS

It's easy to find people who are willing to ascribe to supplements the power to cure almost any ailment including migraine, but hard scientific data has been harder to come by. Recently, though, some evidence has been pointing to the value of some of these substances.

Although the use of mega-vitamin therapy has not been demonstrated to be effective in headache treatment, evidence is growing that some vitamins and elements in particular may have value as migraine preventatives.

For example, a study involving 55 people found that those who took large daily doses of vitamin B2, or riboflavin, experienced 37 percent fewer migraines than those who took a placebo during a three-month study, the February 1998 issue of *Neurology* reported.

The vitamin showed the most benefit after two months of daily use and also decreased the number of days the migraines lasted, the study said. The report also said that riboflavin may work best for those with moderate migraines occurring a few times a month. The dosage of riboflavin used—400 mg—must be obtained by prescription, so those wishing to try it should discuss it with their doctor.

Although it is not known why riboflavin is effective, the report speculated that it might be because the vitamin increases the amount of energy found in the body's cells. Studies have found that migraine sufferers have reduced energy reserves between attacks. An earlier study, reported in 1994 in *Cephalalgia*, also pointed to the potential migraine benefits of this vitamin.

In his practice at the New England Center for Headache, Dr. Fred D. Sheftell has found 50 to 100 mg of vitamin B6 and 400 units of Vitamin E daily to be of use, but he noted that more research is needed.

Another substance finding favor is the element magnesium. Although it's not universally accepted, there is a belief that magnesium depletion, which is having lower-than-normal amounts of magnesium in your body, may contribute to migraines.

Magnesium influences factors such as serotonin, blood vessel size and inflammation, and therein may lie the connection, believes Alexander Mauskop, M.D., author of *The Headache Alternative: A Neurologist's Guide to Drug-Free Relief*. In an interview, Mauskop, a neurologist who heads the New York Headache Center, said that he's found magnesium to be one of the most effective of the non-drug therapies used in his clinic.

In an article in 1995 in the journal *Neurology*, Mauskop demonstrated that the intravenous use of magnesium could relieve migraine. There is evidence that magnesium supplements may also be useful. In research published in 1996 in the journal *Cephalalgia*, magnesium supplements were given to eighty-one men and women who suffered from an average of three to four migraines a month. The study, which compared those taking the supplements to those who were given a placebo, found those who took the supplements experienced significantly fewer migraines.

However, definitive proof of the magnesium connection is not yet in, due to the absence of large-scale, double-blind trials. Still, as Mauskop notes in his book, these smaller studies suggest that having an adequate amount of magnesium in your diet may help prevent migraine.

What's the best way to beef up your daily intake of magnesium?

First, add foods which are rich in magnesium to your diet. The government's Recommended Daily Allowances recommend that men consume 280 mg and women 350 mg of magnesium daily. Foods rich in magnesium include wheat bran, whole grains, dark green leafy vegetables, meats, nuts, beans, milk and bananas.

Obviously, you may recognize some of these foods listed later in this book as migraine triggers. If you're sensitive to them, you might want to opt for a magnesium supplement. If you do, stick to dosages that are similar to the R.D.A. requirements.

Dr. Mauskop also recommends that the magnesium supplement you choose be of the slow-release variety, as many magnesium supplements are poorly absorbed by the body and some can cause diarrhea.

If you do opt for a magnesium supplement, be careful about taking higher-than-recommended dosages. Magnesium can cause drowsiness, weakness and lethargy, and severe overdoses can result in serious health problems and even death. People with kidney disorders, particularly the elderly, are vulnerable to toxic liver effects.

Substances such as riboflavin, magnesium and others may turn out to be effective tools in migraine prevention. In the meantime, discuss with your doctors which ones are right for you.

PART SIX

MIGRAINE-PROOF YOUR LIFESTYLE

#36

IDENTIFY YOUR MIGRAINE TRIGGERS

One of the most fascinating—and infuriating—things about migraines is their capricious nature. Attacks seem to come on for no known reason. But sometimes there is a pattern that can be discerned. This is where the notion of migraine triggers comes in.

Migraine triggers are factors, such as certain foods, or certain environmental conditions, that can be linked to migraine. With our increased understanding of the biology of migraine, these factors are no longer believed to cause attacks; they are believed to "trigger" them in people who are prone to getting migraines in the first place.

During an attack, after all, most migraineurs are exceedingly sensitive to light, sound, and even touch. The physical action of walking down stairs can worsen a migraineur's pain. It's not surprising, then, that migraineurs are more sensitive to their surroundings, the foods they eat, changes in weather, and other factors than those who are migraine-free.

In some migraineurs, light seems to trigger migraines. This

can include bright, flashing, or flickering lights. Steve, for example, can't abide a camera flashlight going off in his face. Heather finds that, if she forgets her sunglasses, bright sunlight can trigger a migraine.

A study published in 1994 in *Headache* looked at 1,044 female migraineurs and found that those whose attacks were set off by visual triggers, such as glare, flicker, patterns, or colors, tended to be those who experienced migraine with aura. They also experienced more severe and incapacitating migraines. The study also found that the participants most vulnerable to these visual triggers were between the ages of forty and sixty.

It's only common sense that loud, continual noise, like that of a pneumatic drill, could not help but trigger a headache in most people. Other people, though, are sensitive to lesser amounts of noise, like that from household appliances, or the noise of a crowd. For some people, odors, aromas, or smells can trigger a migraine. This can include odors from paint, cleaning compounds, cooking odors, perfumes, factory fumes and air pollution.

Stress is also considered a migraine trigger. That complex topic was discussed above.

Generally, migraine triggers fall into these categories:

- Dietary—various foods and food additives
- Environmental—bright lights or glare; loud noises; strong odors; changes in temperature, weather, humidity or altitude; tobacco smoke
- Behavioral—stress, anger, resentment, depression, anxiety and fatigue
- Activity—the motion from riding on trains, planes, automobiles, and bikes, lack of sleep, too much sleep, eyestrain, a fall or head injury
- Hormonal factors—the menstrual cycle, replacement estrogen, oral contraceptives

- Medications—as noted earlier, while the overuse of over-the-counter and prescription pain relievers do not technically create migraine, they can cause rebound headaches. Certain prescription medications—such as nitroglycerin and some high blood pressure medications—can cause headaches.

How big a part do these triggers play in migraine? A group of researchers at the University of Mississippi Head Pain Center in Jackson, are seeking to answer this question.

According to their research, presented in 1997 at the Thirty-ninth Annual Scientific Meeting of the American Association for the Study of Headache, migraineurs pointed to behavioral and environmental factors as the predominant triggers of their headaches, with hormonal and dietary factors relegated to a lesser role. The researchers queried fifty-six clinic patients about their migraine triggers. Triggers cited included stress and worry, lack of sleep or too much sleep, skipping meals, and environmental factors such as glaring lights, strong odors, cigarette smoke, and weather changes.

But migraine triggers aren't always that easy to pin down, warns Dr. Roger Cady, director of the Headache Care Clinic in Springfield, Missouri. He prefers to term them risk factors, because the word *trigger* gives the impression that each time a person is exposed to one of these factors, a migraine will result. For some people, this is true, but for many others, it isn't.

In addition, sometimes you'll be more sensitive to a particular trigger. Karen, for example, is able to eat hot dogs without any problem except when her period is due. If she eats them then, she'll get a migraine.

Furthermore, since the list of potential migraine triggers is so long, it's virtually impossible to have a few days go by without being exposed to one. So if you think back to a few days before your migraine, you can almost always find a suspect trigger, but it may be impossible to determine whether or not it caused the migraine or was just coincidence.

Since there are many potential migraine triggers, trying to ferret out yours can be a lengthy process. But if you can discover your migraine triggers, eliminating them can go a long way in reducing your attacks.

#37

KEEP A MIGRAINE CALENDAR

One of the most valuable tools in dealing with migraine doesn't necessarily come from a doctor's office or pharmacy; you create it yourself using a simple notebook. Some people call it a migraine diary, others a migraine calendar. The name doesn't matter; what is essential is that you use it to record your migraines as well as all the factors that may influence them.

A migraine calendar is designed to record the aspects of your life that pertain to your migraines. It also includes any drug treatments and lifestyle changes you make. Women should include details about their menstrual cycle to gauge the role that hormones may play.

You should keep such a record for at least three months, but many migraineurs find it useful to keep an ongoing calendar. They use it to keep track of their migraines and whether treatment is helping. Obviously, if you are in the midst of a migraine attack, writing is probably the last thing you'll want to do, but you can fill in the record as soon as possible afterward.

Some people find it essential to keep very detailed logs. John, for example, is a fifty-year-old computer programmer whose migraines began eleven years ago. For the past seven years, he has kept a very detailed, ongoing log that is divided into the following four categories:

- Food. This includes everything that John eats and drinks, broken down by ingredients. Such detailed accounting has enabled John to discover his sensitivity to certain ingredients, including food additives.
- Weather. In this section, John records the temperature, barometric pressure, and humidity.
- Migraine attacks and the treatments he's used. Keeping such a record has enabled John to discover the least amount of medication he needs to take that will still be effective.
- Miscellaneous. Any other factors, such as activities he did the day before an attack.

Judi, who has a long history of migraines, also has found keeping a calendar useful.

First, she uses a drug calendar to keep track of all the drugs she takes, including when she took them and, if she needed more, when that was and the amount she used.

She also used a calendar to discover her food triggers. She kept track for a year of all the foods on typical "trigger lists" (such as the one later in this book), but she kept track of other foods she ate as well.

"By using the calendar, I learned that I can eat cheese, chocolate, and peanut butter, but look out for coconut, lima beans, and Brussels sprouts," she said. She also found she was sensitive to exotic fruits, like guava and passion fruit.

Judi uses a calendar to keep track of other facets of her life as well.

"I take note of the barometric pressure before a rainstorm.

From the notes on my calendar, I realized that I had been sensitive to these pressure drops for years but hadn't made the connection. I also learned to be very careful on vacations to hot places, because I now know I get migraines in hot climates," she notes. She also keeps a calendar to note how stress, such as family deaths, affects her migraines.

How much detail you wish to keep depends on you. If you're just beginning to think about your migraine triggers, more detail may be needed; if you're a veteran, less. Says Leah, who has suffered from migraines for twenty-three years, "Most people who have regular migraines will have a light bulb in their head switch on when they review a list of possible triggers and realize, 'Oh, yeah, that's what happens to me.' "

Here are some tips on creating your own migraine calendar.

Use a notebook. In it, include:

- The date and time of the migraine
- How long it lasted (including any preheadache, aura, or postheadache phase)
- The level of pain on a scale of one (mild), two (moderate), and three (severe)
- Any other symptoms (nausea, vomiting, diarrhea)
- Any sensitivities you felt, such as an intolerance to light and noise

In addition, you should include any medications (over-the-counter and/or prescription), including the name of the medicine, when you took it, how much you took, and whether it worked or not, again using a scale ranging from zero (for none) to one (slight relief) to two (moderate) to three (complete).

Also record the possible triggers you experienced within forty-eight hours of the attack. This includes recording everything you eat and drink. Many people find it easier, at least in the beginning, to record everything as they consume it; that way they don't have to try to remember every detail afterward. When you do record your food intake, remember to list ingredients, not just the item. You may discover you're sensitive to an ingredient used in a food's processing and not necessarily the food itself.

You should also note other possible influences, including how you slept, the weather, how you traveled, any particular stressors, and other environmental factors. (There's more about these categories later in this book.)

If you are female, it's important to learn whether hormones influence your migraine. Mark the days of your menstrual cycle with an "x."

You can also mark lifestyle changes you've made, such as a physical exercise regimen, relaxation programs, or treatments such as biofeedback or acupuncture. Keeping track of your migraines with your headache calendar will help you evaluate their effect.

#38

MIGRAINE-PROOF YOUR DIET

Although dietary risk factors are blamed for migraines, the facts show that only a minority of sufferers find their headaches are influenced by what they eat. But if you're in that minority—possibly as high as 25 percent—staying away from foods you are sensitive to can make a vast improvement. Sometimes, these associations are easy to spot, and sometimes they're not.

Take Naomi, for example. When she was a child, Saturday was her favorite day of the week because she got to go to the movies, eat chocolate bars, and, to top it off, on Saturday nights, her mom made her favorite food, hot dogs, for dinner. And, recalls Naomi, "every single Saturday night, I'd get a migraine." Every single week. Since then, Naomi's learned that the nitrates in the hot dogs caused her migraines.

Exactly why certain foods increase migraine risk isn't fully understood. Some of these foods, including aged cheese, nuts, yogurt, and alcoholic beverages, contain a naturally occurring substance called tyramine, which can act as a blood vessel constrictor. But why other foods are associated with migraine is not known.

For those who find food triggers make a difference, the change can be remarkable. This is what happened to Shirley, who has been migraine-free for several years.

"I had terrible migraines," she recalls. Then Shirley read a list of migraine food triggers in a book and set about eliminating them from her diet. The headaches vanished. Shirley was so impressed that, to this day, she carries copies of that list to hand out to other migraine sufferers.

Some foods which are known migraine triggers have stronger connections than others. But still the evidence can be contradictory, which only speaks to how frustrating pinning down such triggers can be. Consider chocolate, long suspected of causing migraine.

A study published in the journal *Headache* in 1995 looked at the dietary habits of 577 migraineurs seen at a clinic in England. The study found that, of 429 patients, 16.5 percent reported that their headaches were brought on by cheese or chocolate, and nearly always both.

The English researchers also decided to investigate whether migraine sufferers who believed they were sensitive to chocolate actually were. They gave half of the dozen migraineurs chocolate and the other half carob. Five out of the 12 patients who ate the chocolate suffered a migraine attack, while none of those who ate carob did.

On the other hand, a study published in December 1997 in *Cephalalgia* found different results. For this study, researchers at the University of Pittsburgh Medical Center tried to duplicate the earlier studies by giving sixty-three women, half of whom were migraine sufferers, samples of either chocolate or carob. The women were also instructed to keep diaries. The results showed that eating chocolate was no more likely to bring on a migraine than was carob.

But, although it can be tricky, some migraine sufferers

have found that foods do indeed trigger attacks. How can you find out if you are sensitive to certain foods? One way is to try eliminating from your diet the ones you suspect, one at a time, for two weeks. Then, reintroduce the food, eating a lot of it. Notice if there is any change in your headache pattern. Remember, though, experiment with just one food at a time—otherwise you'll get hopelessly confused.

You may find that a certain food does seem to play a role in your headaches, even though it's a small one. Is it worth eliminating this food from your diet? That's a call you'll have to make.

You also may discover that certain foods only bother you some of the time. Some women who get migraines around the time of their period sometimes find certain foods make them worse. Of, if you suspect a migraine may be coming on, avoiding your dietary risk factors can help. This is true for Sheila, who has learned to recognize that, when she's about to get a migraine, she'd best steer clear of her dietary triggers. "If I feel like my head is expanding, and my nose gets congested, I know I'm getting a migraine. If I eat pizza laden with cheese, I'll get it for sure. So I eat fruits and vegetables instead and sometimes I avoid the migraine completely."

In their books on migraine, Drs. Alan Rapoport and Fred Sheftell recount some of the common dietary risk factors. Some are elaborated on later on in this book.

- Caffeine and caffeinated foods and drink, such as coffee, tea, chocolate, cocoa, colas and other soft drinks containing caffeine
- Alcoholic beverages
- Dairy products, particularly those which are aged or fermented, like sour cream and yogurt, or aged cheese
- Foods high in yeast, such as doughnuts, coffee cake, and freshly baked bread
- Processed meats which contain the chemical nitrate

This list includes bologna, salami, pepperoni, bacon, ham and hot dogs.

- Vegetables—Some types of beans (broad, Italian, lima, lentil, fava, soy), sauerkraut, onion, peas
- Chocolate (remember, the studies are conflicting, so chocolate hasn't necessarily been exonerated for everyone)
- Sugar and products which contain sugar or corn syrup
- Citrus fruits in large quantities, as well as bananas and figs
- Pork, game, and organ meats, including liver, sweetbreads, kidney and brains
- Food additives, especially monosodium glutamate (MSG)

Lists of other known migraine triggers include nuts, peanuts, peanut butter, pickles, seeds, sesame, other fruits, including avocado, raisins, papaya, passion fruit, red plums, raspberries, plantains, pineapples; and licorice candy. In addition, aspartame, the widely used sweetener sold under the names of Nutrasweet and Equal, has been listed as a migraine trigger. Aspartame, like MSG, is found in a wide array of processed and prepared foods.

Shirley found she had to eliminate many foods from her diet to stay migraine-free but decided it was worth it. You may not need to take such a drastic measure but, by trial and error, can determine—and eliminate—the food causing the problem.

#39

Don't Overuse Caffeine

Ever since our forefathers tossed boxes of tea overboard in Boston Harbor, we've been an enthusiastic nation of coffee drinkers. We're hooked on coffee—and caffeine.

Legend holds that the pharmacist who invented Coca-Cola syrup did so as a remedy for "sick headache," the name commonly used for migraine back then. Caffeine is known for its pain-relieving benefits. Many migraineurs know that a cup of strong coffee can make an impending attack disappear, and caffeine is found in many pain relievers.

So what's the problem? Caffeine is a double-edged sword. While it doesn't give you headaches, if you are accustomed to drinking it and go without, you may very well experience a withdrawal headache.

In a paper published in the February 1997 issue of *Neurologic Clinics,* Fred D. Sheftell, M.D., discusses the complex relationship between caffeine and headache. His concern isn't necessarily the caffeine but the vast quantities of it we Americans consume.

According to Dr. Sheftell, it's been found that more than 85 percent of Americans consume about two hundred milligrams of caffeine daily on average. But often it can be more—a lot more. At his headache clinic, the New England Center for Headache in Stamford, Connecticut, Dr. Sheftell finds it isn't unusual for patients to report they consume five or more cups of coffee per day. "When the staff inquires, 'Cups or mugs?' the answer is invariably mugs," he writes, adding that a mug may equal two to three five-ounce cups. And coffee isn't the only way to get caffeine; it's found in tea, chocolate, and many soft drinks, especially colas.

As noted, if your body is accustomed to caffeine, going without it leads to withdrawal headache. A study published in 1992 in *Cephalalgia* that looked at 151 patients found that 69 percent of those who suffered from "weekend headaches" were those who had a heavy daily caffeine habit and who slept quite late, probably missing their morning dose. Those who used moderate caffeine and woke up earlier didn't experience this type of headache.

Think about your daily routine. If you go without coffee, and a headache kicks in eighteen to thirty-six hours after your last cup, that's an indication your headache may actually be due to caffeine withdrawal. And if your headaches occur on the weekends, after you've missed your "first thing in the morning" cup of coffee, that's another clue.

Although it doesn't take long to rid your body of caffeine, the withdrawal headache can last from four to ten days. So if it's been several days since your last cup of coffee, and you're still getting headaches, you might easily assume it's from something else, when the coffee is still to blame.

Is being dependent on a morning cup of coffee necessarily a problem?

Not necessarily. Despite all the studies that have been done, caffeine has been exonerated from causing any health problems. But since it's a stimulant, some people are sensitive to its effects and find that it causes heart palpitations or makes them feel jittery. If this is true in your case, you may want to reduce your caffeine intake. To accomplish this without inviting a withdrawal headache, Dr. Sheftell recommends a very gradual tapering-off of caffeine intake, such as reducing the amount of coffee you drink by five ounces every five to seven days, until you succeed in discontinuing it or reach a low-maintenance dose of 100 to 120 milligrams per day.

Usually, it's easiest to kick caffeine by weaning yourself off it. But if this doesn't help, discuss the problem with your doctor, who can give you medications to help you deal with the effects of caffeine withdrawal.

Whether or not caffeine is a problem for you is your individual decision, but if you do use caffeine, you should take steps to avoid withdrawal headaches.

#40

DRINK ALCOHOL WISELY

Although not all migraineurs are sensitive to its effects, alcohol is one of the most common migraine triggers. This shouldn't be surprising; headache, after all, is a common hangover symptom. But the effect of alcohol on migraine is more specific than that.

Consider a study published in 1995 in the journal *Headache*. This study, which looked at the drinking habits of 577 patients at an English headache clinic, found that alcohol was more likely to bring on a migraine than a tension headache.

Exactly how alcohol can trigger migraine isn't fully understood, but one possible effect is that alcohol causes the blood vessels to widen, possibly setting off a migraine. But this isn't the whole story, because some types of alcohol are more migraine inducing than others. Studies have shown that wine, particularly red wine, and beer tend to be the worst offenders.

Since red wine appears to be one of the most common of the alcoholic triggers, researchers in England tried to pin down exactly how this substance might affect the brain chemistry.

They gave red wine to both migraineurs and non-migraine sufferers. Their research, published in 1996 in the journal *Cephalalgia*, found no difference in how the red wine affected the brain chemistry of either group.

But, although it's not known exactly how alcohol triggers migraine, it has been found that different types of alcohol affect migraine sufferers differently.

This isn't to say that, if you get migraines, you can't drink alcohol. The study also found that over a quarter of the study's participants could drink any type without getting a migraine. Still, the study found that migraineurs who were sensitive to certain foods were more likely to be sensitive to alcoholic drinks as well.

Generally speaking, the clear liquors, such as gin, vodka and white wine, are less likely to provoke migraines. But, as with anything related to migraine, what is generally true isn't always the case for everyone.

If you find that alcohol triggers a migraine in you, and you can give it up completely, that's fine. If it's less clear that it's a migraine trigger, or if your triggers involve only certain types of liquors, than practice "smart substitutions," suggests Dr. Roger Cady. "We try to teach people 'smart substitutions' because we're living in a culture where having alcohol in moderation is part of the culture," he notes. Choosing white wine if red gives you migraine, for example.

Also, if you are at an occasion where you decide to drink, you should also keep these guidelines in mind:

- Drink as little as possible and slowly.
- Avoid eating any foods that you know cause migraine in you.
- Avoid staying out too late, drinking instead of eating, or doing things that otherwise interrupt your routine.
- Be conscious of "environmental risk factors" that can

bring on migraines in you, such as cigarette smoke or perfume. If the room you're in is smoky, go outside for fresh air.

Much of our culture revolves around social drinking. If alcohol causes migraines for you, and you can give it up, that's best. But, if not, try these guidelines to imbibe more wisely.

#41

BE FESTIVE, NOT FOOLISH

Throughout the year, Susan is bothered only occasionally by migraine attacks. But she gets a whole series of them around Christmas. She used to assume they were caused by the stress of the holiday season. She found this odd, though, because she really enjoys the holidays.

One year, she decided to use her migraine calendar to keep track of the foods she was eating. The mystery was solved.

"I'm normally pretty careful about what I eat at home, but during the weeks between Thanksgiving and New Year's, my office turns into a big party. Everyone brings in trays, people send over baskets of goodies, and it's nonstop gorging," she says. Susan's office parties featured a smorgasbord of goodies found on her personal migraine trigger lists, including red wine, chunks of aged cheese, nuts, and cured meats. These were items that Susan only enjoyed at holiday time.

Holidays can be a dangerous time for some migraineurs, depending on what your particular triggers are. Parties expose you to cigarette smoke and perfume. The alcohol flows freely, and the music can be loud, all of which can bring on an attack.

The stressful preparations involved in the holidays can also help trigger migraines. Although stress doesn't cause migraines, some people find it can act as a trigger or result in tension headaches as well. During the holidays there's always too much to do and too little time. Women especially may face an unfair burden. Nowadays they usually must not only hold down a job but also organize a memorable family celebration, host holiday dinners, make sure all the gifts are bought and wrapped, the cards addressed and sent, and even the stocking hung for the family dog!

Here are some tips to keep your holidays migraine-free:

- If your doctor will be away for the holidays, make sure you have enough migraine medication on hand.
- If the noise, crowds, music, and bright lights of shopping malls bring on a migraine for you, do your shopping from catalogs or in less crowded museum stores.
- Sit down with your family and negotiate their share of the work. Make a list of holiday chores and let them choose the ones they'd most like to do.
- Don't do everything yourself. Consider hiring a cleaning service or carpet cleaners, or call in a caterer to make some of the food. (Make sure the cleaning items they use or the foods they prepare don't include your migraine triggers.) You may want to hire serving help as well. That way, the party is cleaned up as it progresses and you're not faced with a mess the next morning.
- Make sure you have migraine trigger–free goodies on hand and serve either alcohol that won't trigger a migraine or an alcohol-free punch.
- Make sure that you keep your house smoke-free. If you know ahead of time that a guest may wear perfume, and you are sensitive to it, speak up. No friend would want to inadvertently make you suffer.

- Give yourself some time to gently unwind after the holiday season.
- Above all, remember that perfection is a myth. Those beautiful Norman Rockwell holiday paintings are just that—paintings. Real life isn't perfect, and real families and holidays aren't either.

If you're the guest, not the host, here are some additional tips for enjoying the festivities:

- Avoid alcoholic punches, including eggnog. Even if you're not sensitive to certain types of alcohol, a mixed brew can include ingredients that may trigger an attack. If you drink, do so in moderation. What migraineur wants a hangover headache? Eat something first; foods high in fructose (such as fresh fruit) can help you metabolize the alcohol.
- Watch out for unidentifiable appetizers or mystery entrees. Common migraine triggers like cold cuts and dips are often served and you'll have no way of knowing their ingredients.
- Even if you're counting calories, don't skip meals before a party. In addition to bringing on a migraine, being too hungry can cause you to eat foods that you shouldn't.
- If loud music bothers you, ask the host to turn it down a little, or seek out another room.
- If you feel an attack coming on, take your medication and seek out some quiet.
- Don't stay up too late.

#42

Be a Weather Watcher

A stretch of gray weather may seem dreary to most people, but for Terri the day the weather changes, giving way to blue skies and sunshine, signals her impending migraine. "When the weather is beautiful, that's when I think, 'Oh, no,'" she says.

Indeed, changes in weather, which bring rises and dips in barometric pressure, spell trouble for many migraineurs. Although it's not certain why weather affects migraineurs in such ways, apparently changes in air pressure act on the blood vessels in the brain in such a way as to induce attacks. Migraineurs have this sensitivity to weather in common with people who suffer from sinus headaches, and this similarity might account for some of the confusion between the two conditions.

Which type of weather patterns bring on attacks? John Michael Coleman, executive director of M.A.G.N.U.M., points to a Canadian study that found that the weather pattern that most commonly causes migraine is the type with these characteristics:

- A drop in barometric pressure
- The passing of a warm front
- High temperature and humidity
- (Sometimes) rain.

According to the study, other problematic patterns included a southeast wind and extreme changes in barometric pressure heralding the changing of weather patterns.

Bitter cold or unseasonable warmth can also sometimes play havoc with migraineurs as well. Humidity is also known to be a trigger, which doesn't surprise Sheila, who began getting migraines only a few years ago, when she lived in Connecticut. These were mild attacks, though, consisting primarily of visual symptoms, without head pain or nausea. When she moved to Kentucky, her migraine attacks got much worse. "I recognized that the humidity was the problem, so I stopped going for walks or exercising outside," she recalls. Her migraines didn't improve, though, until she moved back to Connecticut.

Sunshine is another problem for migraineurs. Although sunshine probably affects migraineurs differently from barometric pressure, the warmth of the sun on the head or the light from it shining in the eyes can bring on migraines in many. This glare from sunlight can occur not only in the summer but in the winter as well, especially as sunlight is reflected off snow. Having the sun in your eyes when you drive can also bring on a migraine.

It would seem that the problem with being sensitive to the weather is that you can't do anything about it. But that's not really true. There are steps you can take that can help. Here are some suggestions:

- If you know a weather change is on the way, take your migraine medication to ward off an attack.
- If you're in a weather pattern that induces a migraine,

be careful to avoid any of your other migraine triggers during this time.

- If you're sensitive to humidity, avoid sources of steam, such as hot tubs, hot baths, saunas, and steam baths. Using an air conditioner may also help.
- If you're sensitive to sunlight, be aware of the time you spend out in the sun, wear sunglasses, stay in the shade, wear a hat, and use the visor in your car. If you can, adjust your schedule so you won't be driving with the sun in your eyes.
- If you're traveling to a location where the weather is different—for example, more humid or warm—take along your migraine medication. If necessary, take some ahead of time.
- Be careful when you visit high altitudes. Because of the lower level of oxygen in the air, blood vessels expand to compensate, and a migraine may result.

#43

MIGRAINE-PROOF
YOUR WORKPLACE

Ergonomics, the applied science of the workplace, looks at how the workplace can be designed to maximize productivity by reducing worker fatigue and discomfort. If you get migraines at work, there may be some aspect of the ergonomics of your office or workplace that could be improved.

Look around your office. Do you work in a building with sealed windows and poor ventilation? Poorly ventilated rooms cause headaches in some people. The unclean air that causes "sick building syndrome" can cause headaches as well as other problems. Do your coworkers wear perfume? These conditions can trigger migraine attacks.

What about the light? Inadequate lighting can lead to eyestrain, which can cause migraine in some people. But fluorescent lights can be a problem as well. Although you don't realize it, these lights are constantly flickering and can set off migraines as well. Replacing them with conventional bulbs may help.

If you work at a computer, is the screen the proper height so that you are not straining your neck? Taking a break is particularly important if you work at a computer or must perform other types of repetitive movement.

Eyestrain is also a problem for those who do computer work. Take five-minute breaks every one to two hours and, if possible, move to another part of the room where the lighting is different. Look off into the distance or close your eyes and give yourself a brief break from the computer screen.

Do you practice proper posture at your desk? Sit with your back straight and your feet firmly planted on the floor. Make sure your office furniture is designed with your body in mind.

There's a larger issue involved as well. Even if there are aspects of your workplace that may bring on migraine, you may be reluctant to speak up. You may be afraid of being fired or considered a malingerer. In the minds of many, getting migraines is still linked with an inability to handle stress, so you may be afraid of jeopardizing your chances for promotion. Or you may be concerned that other workers will construe your concerns as demands for special privileges.

Laura understood these issues all too well. As a designer, Laura worked in a glass-enclosed office, with her table facing directly into the sun. Knowing that sunshine triggered her migraines, she spoke up and asked for window shades. Her coworkers, who appreciated the light-filled environment, were not enthusiastic. But Laura was able to arrange the shades so that their sunlight was only minimally affected. "People were upset at first, but they later came to understand that I really needed this change to be able to work without pain," she said. But sometimes bosses and coworkers are not this understanding.

If you are faced with such a situation, you may need to make your boss or supervisor aware that your rights as a migraineur are protected by the 1990 Americans with Disabilities Act (ADA). In the case of migraineurs, this federal law offers several protections. For instance, the law requires all employers over a certain size to make "reasonable accommodations" to keep workers with disabilities on the job. This might mean providing you with a flexible work schedule, an area where you can lie down if you sense a migraine attack is coming on, or modifications in office furniture or lighting. Sometimes making your employer aware of this law will be sufficient. (See Chapter 48 for more information.) If you need to obtain further information, contact M.A.G.N.U.M., which is listed in the Resources section.

If you are seeking changes in your workplace, remember it's sometimes better to discuss the problem in a friendly way and offer solutions, not just find fault. For instance, if the fluorescent lights in your office trigger attacks, offer your employer scientific information and explain how this change will help you be more productive.

In the event that your migraines are so severe they prevent you from holding a job, you may be entitled to Social Security disability benefits. (For more information, see Chapter 48.)

#44

Be Routine

"The last time I got a migraine was right before my manuscript was due. I stayed up late nights to finish it, got up long before my alarm clock rang, and was conscious of the passing time. The next thing I knew, 'Bam,' there was the migraine," recalls Alex, who is a novelist.

Nobody likes to be a party pooper, but many migraineurs find that sticking to a routine can be very beneficial. As noted earlier, migraineurs tend to be sensitive to change.

In the course of our daily life, we're often pressured to vary from our routine. Urgent work deadlines pile up, and you have to be in the office early (skipping breakfast), work through lunch, or stay late at your desk (skipping dinner). There are also some more tempting reasons to vary your routine. The holiday parties bring with them ample opportunities to stay out too late. An old friend drops by and wants to go out on the town. Or you may not want to disappoint your spouse by calling it an early night, or you may want to not look like a wet blanket in front of a date.

Remember, though, you have a right to keep the hours you feel are best for you. If you had a more visible disease, people would look out for your welfare. As a migraineur, it's up to you to set the schedule which works for you, and to safeguard your health.

An important aspect of keeping a healthy routine is eating regular meals. You may find such advice old-fashioned; after all, in these hectic times, the best many of us can do is grab a snack. But skipping meals can result in tension headaches. If you get migraines, additional headaches are not something you need!

Some researchers believe that hypoglycemia is linked to migraine. If you are hypoglycemic, which means your blood sugar level can dip too low, you probably know this can cause you to become dizzy or result in a headache. But even those who aren't hypoglycemic make their bodies work overly hard by skipping meals. Such changes in blood sugar can precipitate a migraine attack.

Many migraine experts say it's important to eat a nutritious breakfast. If you're not hungry in the morning, try a bagel and juice. Your body needs fuel to function and, if you become too hungry, that can set the stage for a migraine. If you eat on the run, you may be tempted to stoke up on fast food, which is laden with ingredients that can be migraine triggers.

Even though you should eat regularly, this doesn't have to be the "three square meals" we were taught. Some people find that their blood sugar is kept more even by "grazing," or eating several small, nutritious meals throughout the day. You are the best judge of the eating schedule which is right for you.

#45

Travel with Care

For most migraineurs, the worst time for a migraine to strike is during travel. Unfortunately, that's when it often does. Confinement in a small space, changes in air pressure, exposure to tobacco smoke, the hassles of trying to make a plane or a train are all factors that can combine to cause an attack.

Here are some tips that can help:

- If you're female and you're subject to menstrual migraines, don't schedule your trip around the time you're expecting your period, if possible.
- Tuck an extra supply of your medication in your handbag or carry-on luggage. That way, you can have it handy if you need it, and you don't have to worry about your suitcase getting lost and having to retrieve it. Also bring along written copies of your prescriptions.
- Request your seat ahead of time. If being confined is stressful for you, request an aisle seat. Remember to get up and walk about during the flight.

- Leave for the airport in plenty of time to avoid a last-minute, stressful rush to the plane.
- If you have an early morning flight, or if you're getting in late, consider staying in a hotel near the airport before or after you travel. Make sure that the hotel isn't noisy, or pack some ear plugs, so you'll get a good night's sleep.
- Adhere to your routine. Too often, if you're getting ready for a trip, you may forget about this and stay up too late getting ready or skip meals.
- If you're changing time zones, keep your watch set on your time back home and, if possible, adhere to your normal sleeping and waking times.
- Carry some healthful snacks with you. Remember that the days of in-flight meals and substantial snacks are gone, and the snacks that are handed out, like peanuts, can cause problems for some migraineurs.
- Don't strain your neck and shoulders by carrying heavy luggage. Use a cart or hire an airport porter to carry the extra load.
- Carry that letter from your doctor, mentioned earlier, that attests to your condition as a migraine patient. The letter should spell out the diagnosis as well as the treatments needed if you have to seek emergency treatment in your new destination.
- Turn down your flight attendant's offer of alcoholic beverages, but drink plenty of fluids, because flying is dehydrating.
- Bear in mind that motion can, in some people, bring on migraines. If you get motion sick when you travel, ask your doctor for motion sickness medication.

#46

CONSIDER STARTING AN EXERCISE PROGRAM

Gabriel, a twenty-five-year-old meteorologist, finds that pulse-pounding, aerobic exercise can sometimes help her banish a headache. But for Judi the experience has been the opposite.

"My husband and I do like to ballroom dance, and we dance once or twice each week for an evening. Usually this is not intense enough to trigger a headache, but anything like hiking uphill, or running—anything where I breathe hard—causes a migraine within the hour. It's as sure a trigger for me as food with nitrates or cigarette smoke."

Sharon's experience falls roughly in the middle. She runs and swims four or five times a week and works out with weights—but not if she wakes up with a bad migraine. "If the migraine is mild, I do my usual exercise. The pain goes away while I'm exercising and doesn't come back until I've cooled down. But if the migraine is already bad when I wake up, I've learned to skip exercising that day," she says.

Research findings on the effect of exercise on migraine have been mixed. Some studies suggest that aerobic exercise may be beneficial, but other studies have found that vigorous exercise, such as lifting or bending, can bring on a headache, possibly because of changes in the body's demand for oxygen.

A Canadian study published in 1992 in *Headache* found that exercise does appear to help. Eleven migraineurs, and nine people without migraine, participated in a six-week cardiovascular exercise program. All the participants improved their fitness. This study did not prove that exercise can prevent migraine, but those who completed the program said their headaches were less painful and debilitating.

Remember, if you're middle-aged and inactive, and you're just embarking on a vigorous exercise program, check with your doctor. This is especially true if you have risk factors for coronary heart disease. However, almost anyone can become more active safely, even by starting with a brisk, ten-minute walk each day and gradually increasing the amount of activity until you find what works best. You should, though, be aware of certain types of headaches that are associated with exercise.

Exertional Headaches

Some people get these headaches, also sometimes known as sports headaches, when they exercise. In 1994 the British *Journal of Sports Medicine* published a study in which 129 people who get this type of headache were queried. It was found that men primarily got this type of headache from contact sports, while women experienced them more often while running and jogging.

In most people, getting a headache during exercise is harmless and can often be prevented by taking a pain reliever, such as Advil, an hour or so before exercising. And if you find that very intense exercise brings on a headache, opt for a less intense activity, like brisk walking, bicycling, or swimming.

CARDIAC HEADACHE

Occasionally a headache that comes on with exercise can be a warning sign of high blood pressure, even heart disease or an impending heart attack.

The onset of a cardiac headache is similar to that of the chest pain from coronary heart disease, which is pain caused by a lack of oxygen to the heart. This type of headache can occur even in the absence of chest pain. It begins during exercise and is relieved by rest. If you're over forty and you've just started getting headaches like this, and you are at risk for heart disease, your doctor should check this out. Heart disease risk factors are:

- Age (over 40 for men; over 55 for women)
- Family history of heart disease
- High blood pressure
- Diabetes
- Smoking
- Sedentary lifestyle
- Obesity
- Abnormal blood cholesterol levels

SEX HEADACHES

The exertion of having sex can sometimes trigger a headache as well; such headaches can occur in different forms. Sometimes a very intense headache occurs at the moment of climax. One can also have a dull ache that begins during foreplay and builds gradually in intensity. Generally, these headaches subside quickly, although there is also a type that can linger.

Who gets these headaches? Women are five times more likely. These headaches also often, but not always, occur in people who get other types of headaches, including migraines and exertional headaches, according to a study published in 1997 in the *Journal of Neurology, Neurosurgery and Psychiatry.*

It isn't known what causes these headaches. One theory is that it may be the result of straining the nerves of the neck, which may transmit pain to the back of the head, the spinal cord, and brain.

The vast majority of these headaches are harmless; on very rare occasions, though, an intense headache during sex may signal a stroke.

If you are prone to such headaches, ask your doctor about taking propranolol (Inderal) as a preventative. It's believed that this drug may help prevent these headaches by preventing an increase in blood pressure during intercourse.

#47

GET YOUR ZZZZ'S

Many migraineurs complain that they get attacks when they get too little sleep. Many also complain that they can't get a good night's sleep or that they wake up with migraines.

Sleep is a complicated subject. It's difficult to evaluate how much sleep the average person needs. Some of us need less, some more, to feel refreshed; your best guide to how much sleep you need is yourself.

If you suffer from insomnia, this may play a role in your migraines. Almost all of us have an occasional bad night's sleep, when our mind races and we stay awake, despite our best efforts to fall sleep. Experts call this transient insomnia, an annoying but not serious problem. Short-term insomnia is often a problem for people undergoing psychological stress, such as a death, divorce, or job change. If you're suffering from chronic insomnia, which is usually defined as lasting at least three weeks and possibly for months or years, consult your doctor. There may be an underlying problem.

A study published in 1995 in *Headache* looked at twenty-five people who experienced headaches that kept them up at night or were present on their awakening. The study found that some of the people had other problems as well, such as obstructive sleep apnea, which means that they stop breathing for periods while they sleep, a condition which can be life-threatening and should be treated. The study also found that some of the participants who complained of night headaches and insomnia were suffering from rebound headache caused by the overuse of pain relievers. In this case, stopping the medication relieved the headaches and the sleep problems.

Although you may not realize it, you can help guarantee yourself a good night's sleep. Here are some tips:

- Go to bed at the same time each night and awaken at the same time each morning. Do it even on weekends and vacations.
- Use your bedroom only for sleep, not for reading, using your laptop computer, or watching television.
- It's usually better not to take naps during the day unless you're accustomed to doing so. If you do want to nap, make it brief.
- Try physical exercise, like a brisk walk, during the day.
- Reduce your caffeine intake if it makes you too over-stimulated to sleep.
- Reduce your alcohol consumption. Alcohol can make you sleepy, but too much can lead to nightmares.
- Don't smoke at night. Smoking can interfere with the oxygenation of the blood and disrupt sleep.
- Keep your bedroom comfortable. Make sure the temperature is neither too hot nor too cold.
- Keep your bedroom quiet. If you live in noisy surroundings, like near an airport or highway, purchase a device that generates "white noise" to mask the sounds, or play soothing background music.
- Use ear plugs when you travel to block out sounds from

nearby hotel rooms. And if you're concerned about oversleeping when you travel, set the alarm, ask for a wake-up call from the hotel, or both.

- Check your mattress and make sure it is firm. Try a firm pillow rather than a soft one; too-soft pillows can lead to stiffness and headaches as well.

- If you're a woman approaching or in menopause, the hormonal fluctuations you're experiencing may be disturbing your sleep. Consider either replacement hormones or, if they are likely to worsen your migraine, nonhormonal alternatives.

PART SEVEN

Arm Yourself with Information

#48

KNOW YOUR LEGAL RIGHTS

Because migraine is so rarely taken seriously, you may be surprised to learn that you have certain protections guaranteed to you by the federal law known as the Americans with Disabilities Act (ADA). This wide-ranging law was passed by the U.S. Congress in 1990, but its full impact is only now being recognized.

It's generally accepted that this law applies to people who are obviously disabled: those who are physically handicapped, blind, or deaf. These disabilities are easy to see. When it comes to migraine, the application of this law is not that well established. The main reason this law is often not considered when it comes to migraineurs is because migraine is, essentially, an invisible disease.

Invisible to all, perhaps, except the migraineur. You know full well that, if you're in the midst of a migraine attack, you may be unable to think, speak, coordinate your movements, or do much of anything at all. You also may be seized by waves of vomiting and nausea.

If you have mild migraine attacks, those that disable you for perhaps a day or two a month, you may not think of yourself as disabled. But think about it. Are there times when you have hidden your illness from your boss, afraid that you'll be fired or passed over for promotions? And if you get disabling migraines often, being fired, or not being hired in the first place if your potential employer learns of your disease, may be a real possibility.

That's where the law steps in. Under the ADA, you're protected when you apply for a job because the law stipulates that you don't have to answer questions about your health unless they are directly related to your ability to perform your job. The law also bars an employer from firing you because you have a disease.

The law can also affect your working environment. The ADA requires employers of a certain size to make "reasonable accommodations" to enable you to work on the job. For people with physical handicaps, this could mean special chairs, equipment, curb cuts, or elevators. For people with migraines, it could mean a more flexible work schedule, so you can take time off when you have attacks. Or if your migraines are triggered by fluorescent lights, or working in an overly bright office without window shades, you might be able to convince your employer to change the bulbs or add drapes. Certainly you can try to negotiate these items without resorting to the ADA, but it's good to know you have that protection.

Don't expect, though, that your right to these protections will be well understood. Although it's known that the ADA applies to people with invisible disabilities, just how the law works will become clear as individuals win cases based on the legislation.

What if you suffer from such severe migraines that it's become impossible for you to hold a job? Only an estimated 5 percent of migraine sufferers fall into this category. These are people who suffer from a condition known as intractable migraines, which means that their migraines are not relieved by any treatments. In this case, they may be able to win the right to collect Social Security disability payments. This is not welfare; Social Security disability insurance was created to provide a safety net for working people who have become disabled.

This is also an area in which asserting your rights will not be easy. You have to apply for Social Security disability, and the approval procedure is often arduous. But migraineurs are increasingly winning these cases.

For information on how to protect your rights in these areas, contact M.A.G.N.U.M., which is listed in the Resources section.

#49

KNOW YOUR HEALTH CARE RIGHTS

Something else happened that July day when Kristen felt the familiar sensations of nausea and headache—signals that a migraine attack was imminent. As the day progressed, she had begun feeling worse. Around evening, she felt a tingling and a numbness on the left side of her face that soon spread down the left half of her body. She'd never felt this way before. Alarmed, she called her doctor, who instructed her to go to the local hospital's emergency room immediately. After undergoing several tests, the emergency room physician told her she was suffering from "a tension headache or migraine."

Although Kristen was relieved to learn she hadn't suffered a stroke, she was dismayed a few weeks later, when the hospital bill submitted to her insurance company came back stamped "DENIED."

"I was very angry. I pay a lot for health insurance, and this was supposed to be covered," she said. Her insurer finally paid the bill, but only after repeated calls from Kristen, her doctor, and the emergency room physician. Kristen also had to submit and resubmit her insurance forms, and she was even contacted by a bill collector the hospital hired.

In recent years, health insurance companies have been cutting back on costs. This spells bad news for migraineurs, whether they are covered by private health insurance (the traditional indemnity type), health maintenance organizations (HMOs), or other types of managed health care.

The typical problems faced by migraineurs fall into several major categories, notes Michael John Coleman, executive director of M.A.G.N.U.M., which advocates on behalf of sufferers. These problem areas are as follows.

EMERGENCY ROOM VISITS

Unfortunately, since migraine isn't considered by hospitals to be a life-threatening ailment, sufferers may find their insurers refuse to cover emergency room visits. This is a devastating problem for migraineurs who find themselves in the midst of such severe attacks that their home medication is useless, or those who are experiencing the warning signs of stroke or other serious conditions.

Thus far about ten states have passed laws barring insurers from this practice, and federal legislation is being discussed, but the majority of states currently provide no such protection. M.A.G.N.U.M. succeeded in protecting Medicare patients who sought emergency room treatment due to pain and is trying to widen this protection. In the meantime, read your insurance contract carefully and contest your claim if it is rejected. Also contact your state legislature or local insurance regulatory agency.

Another problem with hospital emergency rooms and HMOs is that a person suffering a visible injury, such as a broken arm, or suffering from stomach pains is seen immediately, but the migraineur in the midst of an excruciating attack may be told to come back hours, days, or even weeks later. This is obviously unfair, but your best recourse is to be assertive about your ailment and explain that you need timely treatment. If you acquiesce, you're reinforcing the misperception that migraine isn't an urgent problem.

REFERRALS TO HEADACHE SPECIALISTS OR HEADACHE CLINICS

It is becoming increasingly difficult to get referred to a headache specialist or clinic. If you have traditional indemnity coverage you can refer yourself, but people are increasingly being covered by HMOs. The vast majority of HMOs keep costs down by using a gatekeeper system, which means such referral requests must be approved by your family doctor or internist.

Another problem is that you may be referred to a professional who you don't believe is the best person to deal with your migraines, such as a psychologist who offers counseling as the main treatment. Counseling can be an important adjunct to migraine treatment, but, as it's becoming clear that migraine is a neurological disease, it requires medical treatment. Arm yourself with information (M.A.G.N.U.M. can provide you with some; see the Resources section) and assert your right to get the appropriate treatment.

OTHER UNCOVERED TREATMENTS

Biofeedback, acupuncture, and other treatments may be considered alternative methods and may not be covered by insurers or HMOs. Again, check your policy carefully, but be aware that you may need to pay for such treatments out of your own pocket.

DRUGS

More and more effective drugs are being developed for migraine. Unfortunately, though, many of these drugs, such as sumatriptan, are expensive, and insurers can limit their use. For example, an insurer may limit a monthly prescription to, for example, two doses, when a patient needs the drug far more often. The insurer also may use the prevention of "drug rebound" as an excuse for limiting these drugs. Although drug rebound is a problem, it occurs more often when people are not using or being denied effective abortive medication. In such cases, send a letter not only to the insurer but also to the drug company, alerting them that you are being denied an effective medication. The company may very well investigate the matter.

Remember that no matter whom you're dealing with, it's usually best to be assertive, though not belligerent. Arm yourself with information about the latest scientific findings on migraine, share it, write letters, and empower yourself to get the best medical care. In some cases, it can help to join with others. The next section discusses how you can do this.

#50

JOIN (OR START) A MIGRAINE SUPPORT GROUP

This book encompasses fifty essential things to do if you are a migraine sufferer. For many people, all this may prove more than enough. However, migraines can be a very frustrating problem. And making lifestyle changes can be difficult. You may want more input on how others have responded to certain drugs or alternative treatments.

For all these reasons, a migraine support group can be of great value. Through it, you can share tips on what works for you, keep up to date on new treatments, learn how others deal with migraine triggers, share your successes, and encourage others. You can learn about support groups from the associations listed in the Resources section of this book.

There is also a world of information—literally—on the Internet. Here you can partake in discussions about migraine with people from all over the world. Bear in mind, though, that what you find on the Internet may range from information in the latest professional medical journals to nonscientists hawking unsubstantiated migraine cures. There's a lot of solid information,

but use your best judgment to weed through it all. To begin
your search, check the Resources section for a list of the best
migraine sites on the Internet.

In short, if you're a migraine sufferer, you may sometimes feel alone. You're not. Share your challenges and successes with others.

Resources

Books

American Council on Headache Education, with Lynne M. Constantine and Suzanne Scott, *Migraine: The Complete Guide*, Dell, 1994.

Diamond, Seymour, M.D., with Bill and Cynthia Still, *The Hormone Headache: New Ways to Prevent, Manage and Treat Migraines and Other Headaches*, Macmillan, 1995.

Inlander, Charles B., and Porter Shimer, *Headache: 47 Ways To Stop The Pain*, Walker, 1995.

Mauskop, Alexander, M.D., F.A.A.N., *The Headache Alternative: A Neurologist's Guide to Drug-Free Relief*, Dell, 1997.

Rapoport, Alan M., and Fred D. Sheftell, M.D., *Headache Relief for Women: How You Can Manage and Prevent Pain*, Little, Brown, 1995.

Robbins, Lawrence, M.D., and Susan Lang, *Headache Help: A Complete Guide to Understanding Headaches and the Medicines That Relieve Them*, Houghton Mifflin, 1995.

Associations

American Association for the Study of Headache (AASH)
875 Kings Highway, Suite 200
Woodbury, NJ 08096
(609) 845-0322

The American Council for Headache Education (ACHE)
875 Kings Highway, Suite 200
Woodbury, NJ 08096
(800) 255-ACHE
AASH is an organization for physicians devoted to the scientific study of headache; ACHE provides patient education.

M.A.G.N.U.M.: Migraine Awareness Group: A National Organization for Migraineurs
208 King Street
Alexandria, VA 22313
(703) 739-9384
(703) 739-2432
A nonprofit health care public education organization devoted to spreading awareness about migraine. Unlike the other associations listed here, which provide information on other forms of headache as well, M.A.G.N.U.M. specializes only in migraine issues.

National Headache Foundation
5252 North Western Avenue
Chicago, IL 60625
(800) 843-2256
(312) 878-7725

The Migraine Foundation
120 Carlton Street, Suite 210
Toronto, Ontario
Canada M5A 4K2
(416) 420-4916
24-hour information line: (800) 663-3557

THE INTERNET

Compuserve, America On Line, Prodigy, and other online services have discussion groups known as forums. Some discuss headache within general health forums; others have specific groups devoted to the discussion of headache and migraine.

On the Internet, there are many websites and news groups devoted to the discussion of headache and migraine. Here is a sampling of the best; you can find lots more by using major search engines, such as Yahoo, and typing in the search word *migraine*. Bear in mind that the Internet is an ever-changing virtual universe, and website addresses can change and even disappear.

American Association for the Study of Headache (AASH):
   http://www.aash.org
American Council for Headache Education (ACHE):
   http://www.achenet.org
National Headache Foundation:
   http://www.headaches.org
JAMA Migraine Information Center:
   http://www.ama-assn.org/special/migraine/migraine.htm
M.A.G.N.U.M.:Migraine Awareness Group:
   A National Understanding for Migraineurs:
   http://www.migraines.org
Women's Health Hot Line: This is a general women's health

newsletter edited by this book's author, Charlotte Libov.
http://www.libov.com

ADDITIONAL SPECIFIC TOPICS

Alternative Medicine

Office of Alternative Medicine
National Institutes of Health
Information Center
6120 Executive Boulevard, Suite 450
Rockville, MD 20892
(301) 402-2466
The government's research branch into alternative therapies.
Offers free fact sheets and other information.

Acupuncture and Acupressure

American Academy of Medical Acupuncture
5820 Wilshire Boulevard, Suite 500
Los Angeles, CA 90036
(800) 521-2262
(213) 937-5514

American Association of Acupuncture and Oriental Medicine
50 Maple Place
Manhasset, NY 10030

National Commission for the Certification of Acupuncturists
1424 16th Street, NW, Suite 501
Washington, DC 20036
(202) 232-1404
Administers testing for certification in acupuncture and Chinese herbology. For referrals, send a $3 check for your state directory or a $24 check for the national directory.

Biofeedback

Biofeedback Certification Institute of America
Association for Applied Psychophysiology and Biofeedback
10200 West 44th Avenue, No. 304
Wheat Ridge, CO 80033
(301) 422-8436
(800) 477-8892
Provides information to help you find a certified biofeedback
practitioner.

Chronic Pain Syndrome

American Academy of Pain Management
3600 Sisk Road, Ste. 2-D
Modesto, CA 95356

Depression and Panic Disorder

American Psychiatric Association
1400 K St., NW
Washington, DC 20005
(202) 682-6000

American Psychological Association
750 First Street, NW
Washington, DC 20002
(202) 336-5500

Diet and Nutrition

American Dietetic Association
216 West Jackson Boulevard, Suite 800
Chicago, IL 60606
(312) 899-0040
(800) 366-1655

Exercise

American College of Sports Medicine
P.O. Box 1440
Indianapolis, IN 42606
(317) 637-9200

Herbal Therapy

American Botanical Council
P.O. Box 201660
Austin, TX 78720
Nonprofit organization that offers information about the bene-
fits of herbs and plants.

Relaxation and Stress Management

American Institute of Stress
124 Park Avenue
Yonkers, NY 10703
(914) 963-1200

The Mind/Body Institute
Division of Behavioral Science
New England Deaconess Hospital
185 Pilgrim Road
Boston, MA 02215
Offers relaxation audiotapes.

Stress Management Program
Cleveland Clinic Foundation
Psychology Dept. P-57
9500 Euclid Avenue
Cleveland, OH 44195
Offers audiotaped stress management program.

TMD or TMJ (temporomandibular [jaw] disorders)

National Oral Health Information Clearinghouse
1 NOHIC Way
Bethesda, MD 20892-3500

Yoga

Himalayan Institute of Yoga, Science and Philosophy
RR1, Box 400
Honesdale, PA 18431
(717) 253-5551
(800) 822-4547
Offers catalog of educational materials as well as referrals to classes around the country.

Yoga Journal
2054 University Avenue, Suite 604
Berkeley, CA 94704-1082
(415) 841-9200

INDEX

Depression, 7, 25, 67–71
D.H.E. 45, 39, 92, 95, 109, 111–12
Diamond Headache Clinic, 42, 65
Diamond, Merle, 42, 112
Dichloralphenazone, 90
Diet, changes in, 84, 153–56
Dihydroergotamine Mesylate (D.H.E. 45), 39, 92, 95, 109, 111–12
Disability benefits, 171, 187
Doctor, choosing a, 55–57, 64–66
Doxepin (Adapin, Sinequan), 103
Drugs *see* Medication
Drug Therapy for Headache, 83

Elavil, 100, 101, 103
Electroencephalography (EEG), 62
Eletriptan, 97
Emergency room visits, 110–13, 188–90
Ergostat, 90
Ergotamine, 47, 90, 95
Ergotamine tartrate, 38, 39, 90, 108
Ergotism, 108
Esgic, 108
Estrogen, 36, 39, 41, 42, 50–51
Exam, physical, 61
Excedrin, 108

Exercise, 84, 176–79
Eyestrain, 28

Familial hemiplegic migraine, 12, 24, 77
Fenoprofen calcium (Nalfon), 38
Feverfew, 138–39
Fioricet, 91, 108
Fiorinal, 91, 108
Fluoxetine (Prozac), 69, 71, 104
Food and Drug Administration (FDA), U.S., 9, 46
Food triggers, 24, 25, 153–56
Freitag, Frederick G., 65

Gallagher, R. Michael, 22, 83

Headache, 67, 94, 96, 129, 136, 146, 154, 160, 177, 180–81
Headache:
  cardiac, 178
  causes of, 27–29, 62
  Chronic Daily Headache (CDH), 13–14, 16, 107, 109
  cluster, 13
  migraine *see* Migraine
  mixed headache syndrome, 65
  posttraumatic, 28
  rebound, 29, 65, 90, 106–9
  sex, 178–79